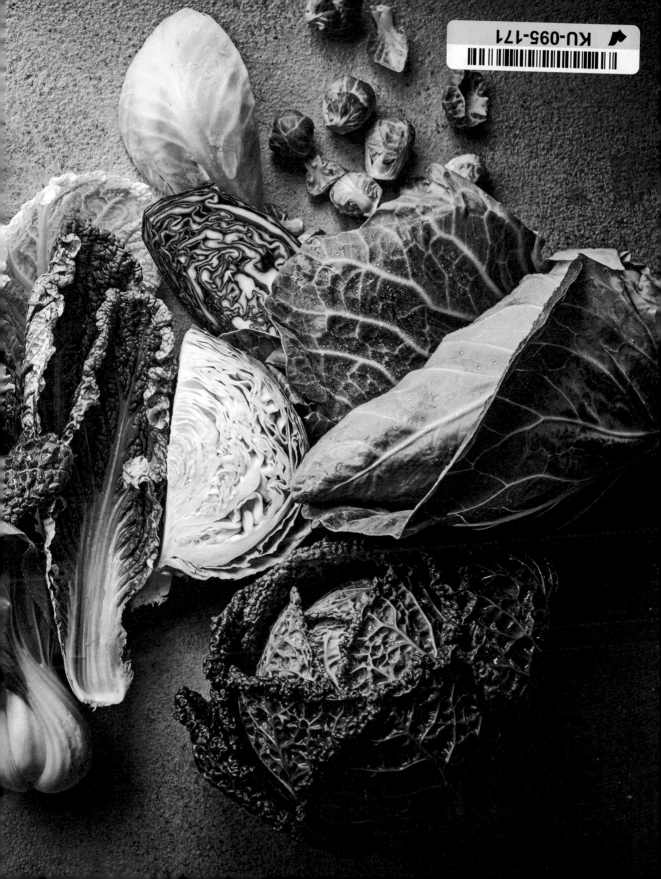

KU-095-171

The Reverse Your Diabetes Cookbook

Lose weight and eat to beat type 2 diabetes

KATIE & GIANCARLO CALDESI
with Jenny Phillips

Photography by Maja Smend

KYLE BOOKS

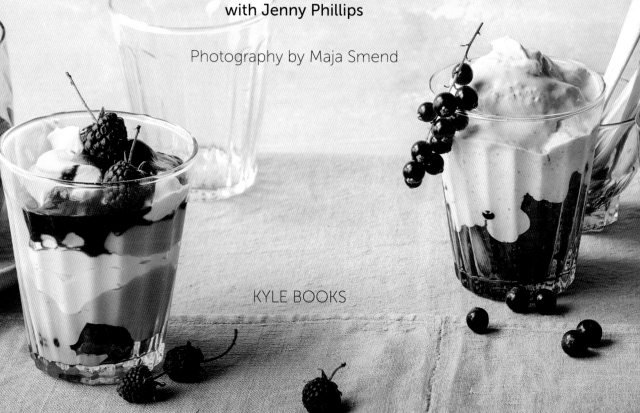

An Hachette UK Company
www.hachette.co.uk

First published in Great Britain in 2020 by
Kyle Books, an imprint of Kyle Cathie Ltd
Carmelite House
50 Victoria Embankment
London EC4Y 0DZ
www.kylebooks.co.uk

ISBN: 978 085783 857 5

Text copyright 2020 © Katie & Giancarlo Caldesi
Photographs copyright 2020 © Maja Smend
Design and layout copyright 2020 © Kyle Cathie Ltd

Distributed in the US by Hachette Book Group, 1290 Avenue of the Americas,
4th and 5th Floors, New York, NY 10104

Distributed in Canada by Canadian Manda Group, 664 Annette St., Toronto, Ontario,
Canada M6S 2C8

Katie & Giancarlo Caldesi are hereby identified as the authors of this work in accordance with
Section 77 of the Copyright, Designs and Patents Act 1988.

All rights reserved. No part of this work may be reproduced or utilized in any form or by any
means, electronic or mechanical, including photocopying, recording or by any information
storage and retrieval system, without the prior written permission of the publisher.

Publisher: Joanna Copestick
Editor: Vicky Orchard
Editorial assistant: Sarah Kyle
Design: Tina Smith Hobson
Photography: Maja Smend
Food and props styling: Susie Theodorou
Production: Allison Gonsalves

A Cataloguing in Publication record for this title is available from the British Library

Printed and bound in China

10 9 8 7 6 5 4 3

Note: The information in this book is only part of how any particular person may decide which diet or indeed lifestyle is the best for them. If you are on prescribed medication or suffer from a significant medical condition we strongly advise you to consult your own doctor before making changes. For example, improvements in lifestyle and weight loss may also significantly improve your blood pressure or diabetes control requiring a reduction in medication. The science part of this book is written from the viewpoint of people with type 2 diabetes or those wishing to lose weight. The recipes may also be suitable for people with type 1 diabetes provided of course that you consult your doctor as advised above. If you are on prescribed medication, it is recommended that you check your plans with your doctor. Type 2 diabetics using insulin may well need advice about a reduction in insulin dosage to avoid the risk of a hypo.

CONTENTS

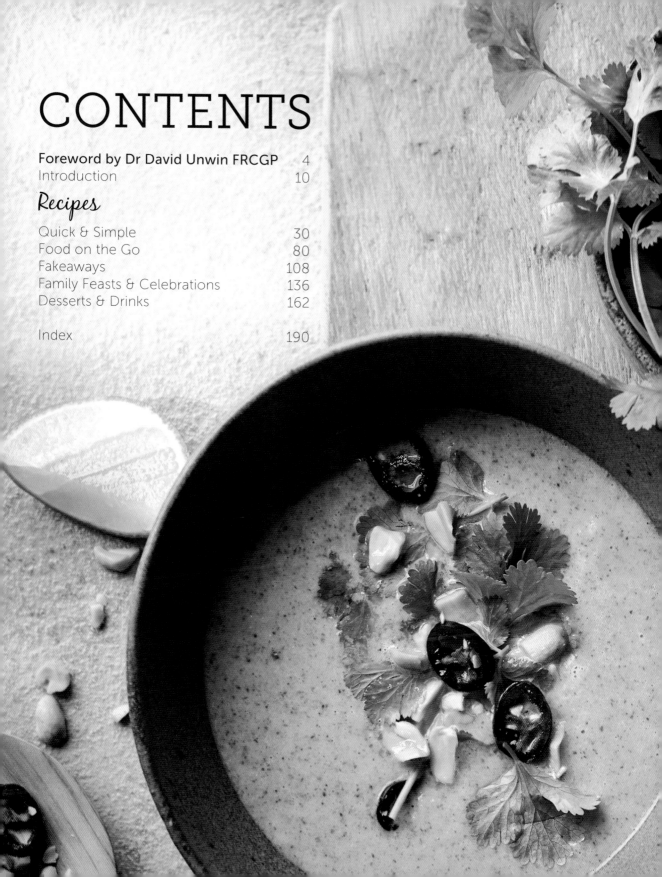

FOREWORD

by Dr David Unwin

Welcome to our second low-carb cookbook.

In *The Diabetes Weight-loss Cookbook*, we described how London chef Giancarlo Caldesi changed his diet to put his type 2 diabetes into remission using recipes devised by his wife Katie. Before I go any further, I should introduce myself and explain my interest in the drug-free treatment of diabetes and other conditions. I am a family doctor based in Southport in the north of England where I have cared for the same population of 9,000 patients since 1986. During this time, I noticed the pressure to prescribe ever-increasing numbers of drugs, and yet many of my patients didn't seem to enjoy good health. An associated problem was the need to add in a second drug to control a side effect caused by the first drug. This felt depressingly like it was trapping my patients into a vicious cycle of polypharmacy. I would give anti-inflammatory drugs to an obese patient with painful knees, but then would have to add in another drug for the side effect of indigestion, and yet another one for the rise in blood pressure, an additional side effect, but then a fourth drug may be needed to counteract the ankle swelling caused by the BP medication. In each case I was failing to address the true cause of illness by applying the sticking plaster of a symptomatic, pharmaceutical remedy. It's entirely possible that a far better route for our hypothetical patient could have been to lose weight in the first place.

Perhaps more relevant to this book is the type 2 diabetes that affected chef Giancarlo so badly that he could no longer feel his feet. My medical model would have been to treat him with the drug metformin, despite the fact that 20 per cent of people taking metformin experience either abdominal bloating or diarrhoea (don't worry, I have extra drugs for that too!) But would metformin deal with the true cause of Giancarlo's diabetes? To put it another way, was his diabetes caused by the failure of his "metformin gland", therefore his treatment

is part of some sort of hormonal replacement? No. Then what is the real cause of his illness? The answer now seems so clear: a sugar – glucose. My older patients still call it "sugar diabetes", which is a pretty good clue. But, embarrassingly, from 1986–2012, although I noticed the epidemic of obesity and an eight-fold increase in the numbers of my patients with type 2 diabetes, it hadn't occurred to me to ask why this should be happening, or whether the situation could be reversed. I saw diabetes as inevitably a chronic, deteriorating condition needing ever-greater doses of medication. This now seems ridiculous and sad. My GP practice has changed, and the day before I sat down to write this piece, I was able to call a patient to tell him that he was the 70th practice patient to achieve drug-free diabetes remission.

Reversing type 2 diabetes

Since writing *The Diabetes Weight-loss Cookbook*, the idea of drug-free reversal of diabetes has really caught the public's imagination. It is an optimistic concept that has given hope to so many. This hope has in turn been the motivation for thousands of people to improve their diet. Not only that, but it is potentially a win-win situation for the National Health Service; every year my GP practice is now spending about £50,000 less on drugs for diabetes than the average for our area.

In clinical practice I prefer to refer to this as putting diabetes into "remission" rather than reversing it, because in reality the condition could easily return if the diet becomes heavy on sugar

"Only yesterday I phoned up a patient with the great news that he was the seventieth practice patient in my care to achieve drug-free diabetes remission."

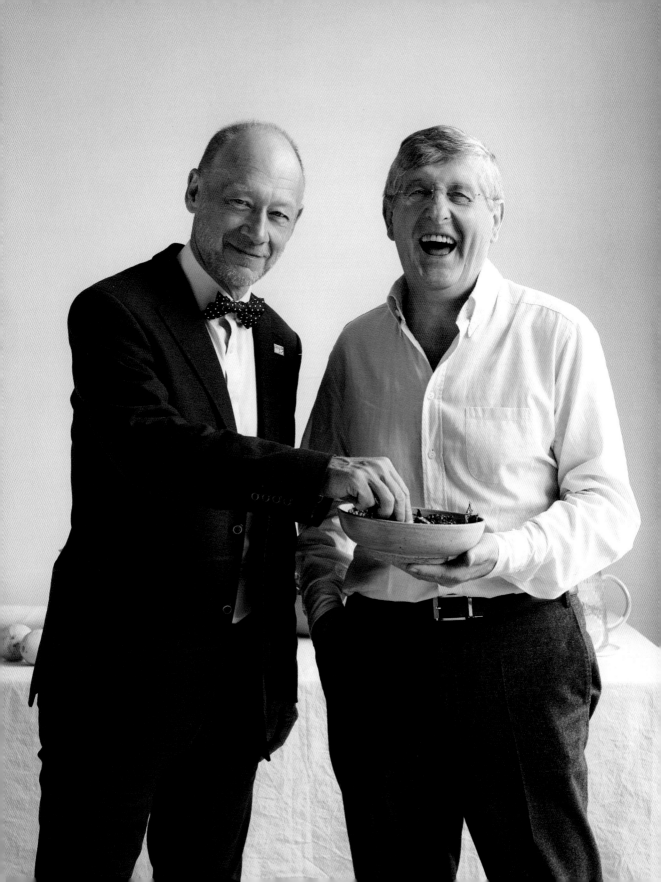

and starchy carbs again. When I give people the choice of starting lifelong medication for diabetes or embracing lifestyle change, 99 per cent are interested in avoiding drugs, just like Giancarlo. To understand how avoiding or reversing diabetes may be possible, let's try to establish what the true cause of this disease could be.

The wonderful professor Roy Taylor, an international expert on diabetes, first helped me to understand the role of a sugar (glucose) and a hormone (insulin) in the development and possible reversal of type 2 diabetes. Insulin is produced by the pancreas gland, and its job is to keep blood sugar low by pushing glucose out of the bloodstream and into cells. In the case of muscle cells, the glucose is a source of energy, but if day after day you consume more glucose than needed for muscular activity (as so easily occurs these days with our sedentary lifestyles), the excess sugar can be pushed into other cells where it is changed into fat.

Three important areas for this are:

● Belly fat, resulting in central or abdominal obesity.
● Liver cells, resulting in a fatty liver (now affecting a worrying 20 per cent of the UK population).
● Pancreas gland cells, where the fat interferes with the production of insulin itself, thereby contributing to diabetes.

Unfortunately, in addition, the fatty liver also interferes with the normal action of insulin, preventing it from working as it should, and resulting in a rise in blood sugar levels. Over time,

unhealthy raised blood glucose levels damage the circulation supplying vital organs (heart, eyes, kidneys), causing many of the consequences of poorly controlled diabetes, including the damaged nerves suffered by Giancarlo.

The good news is that Roy Taylor has shown us that much of this can be reversed, putting diabetes into remission and, in Giancarlo's case, restoring normal blood glucose and the sensation to his feet. I hope you are interested in finding out how this may be achieved. Well, it seems logical to cut off the supply of excess glucose. This can be done in three ways: bariatric surgery, a very low-calorie diet or the subject of this book, a low-carb diet.

How to become a fat burner and less hungry

Nearly all the cells in your body, like the new hybrid cars, are able to burn two different fuels: glucose or fat. However, the higher levels of insulin present in a person eating carbs prevent the use of fat as a fuel. (This explains why I was always hungry for decades, no matter how many biscuits I ate and no matter how much fuel I had stored in my "middle-aged spread".) Going low-carb enabled my metabolism to adjust to fat burning, so I could access the huge reserves of energy in my belly fat and kick-start weight loss where I needed it most. Another aspect of this change in diet was that my ever-nagging hunger vanished in weeks, an outcome that surprises many of my patients.

Given the part glucose plays in diabetes, it seems common sense to stop eating foods that contain glucose. There are three common sources of sugar:

● Naturally sweet foods, such as honey, raisins and bananas.
● Processed foods sweetened with table sugar, including cakes, biscuits and many "low-fat" foods.
● Starchy carbohydrates, for example cereals, potatoes and rice, which are converted into glucose by our digestive system.

Some of you will have heard of the low-GI diet. This refers to the Glycaemic index, a system that ranks carbohydrates in terms of how sugary they are relative to pure glucose, which counts as 100. I used the same glycaemic index to produce a set of infographics to help people understand how foods might affect their blood glucose compared

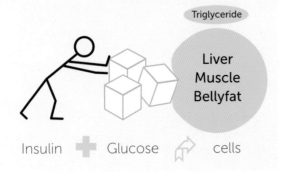

Insulin pushes glucose into the cells where it becomes fatty triglyceride

Triglyceride

Liver
Muscle
Bellyfat

Insulin ✚ Glucose ➭ cells

Three different sources of sugars that make up our total dietary "sugar burden"; shown as 4g teaspoon of table sugar equivalents*

NATURALLY OCCURING SUGARS	FOODS WITH ADDED SUGARS	FOODS CONVERTED INTO SUGAR DURING DIGESTION
Skimmed milk 0.9 teaspoon/100ml (3½oz)	**Fizzy orange (1/3 can)** 1 teaspoon/100ml (3fl ½oz)	**Boiled spaghetti** 3.7 teaspoons/100g (3½oz)
Apple juice 4.3 teaspoons/100ml (3½fl oz)	**Raspberry yogurt** 2.4 teaspoons/100g (3½oz)	**French fries** 5.1 teaspoons/100g (3½oz)
Banana 4.9 teaspoons/100g (3½oz)	**Digestive biscuits** 8.8 teaspoons/100g (3½oz)	**Baked potato** 6.3 teaspoons/100g (3½oz)
Raisins 17.1 teaspoons/100g (3½oz)	**Malt loaf** 14.7 teaspoons/100g (3½oz)	**Basmati rice** 6.8 teaspoons/100g (3½oz)
Honey 17.6 teaspoons/100g (3½oz)	**Chocolate rice snaps** 24.4 teaspoons/100g (3½oz)	**Brown bread** 10.8 teaspoons/100g (3½oz)

* As each food would affect blood glucose, from the international tables of glycaemic index and glycaemic load (Atkinson, Foster-Powell et al., 2008) as per the calculations in a paper published in the *Journal of Insulin Resistance* 'It is the glycaemic response to, not the carbohydrate content of food that matters in diabetes and obesity: The glycaemic index revisited.' D J Unwin et al.

to a teaspoon of sugar (see above). Many people are surprised to learn that a small bowl of rice will raise your blood sugar by the same extent as 10 teaspoons of table sugar. If you have diabetes, pre-diabetes or central obesity, it can make sense to avoid not just sugar but starchy carbs, replacing them with green veg and more protein from meat, fish, dairy products and nuts. This is at the heart of the low-carb diet and the basis for these delicious recipes. My infographics have been endorsed by NICE (The National Institute for Health and Care Excellence) – an advisory body for medical practitioners.

The infographic right explains how a seemingly healthy breakfast of cereals, toast and fruit juice is in fact sugar with sugar and more sugar, in terms of its effect on blood glucose. A better choice for type 2 diabetics would be scrambled eggs and coffee with cream. This would have far higher nutrient density, particularly in terms of protein, while having less than 10 per cent of the effect on blood glucose.

A healthy breakfast?: Cereals, toast & fruit juice

Food item	Serving size	How does each food affect blood glucose compared with one 4g teaspoon of table sugar?
Bran flakes	30g	3.7
Milk	125ml	1
Brown toast (1 slice)	30g	3
Pure apple juice	200ml	8.6
Total for breakfast		16.3

Why this second book?

We have received so much positive feedback from *The Diabetes Weight-loss Cookbook*, but also many suggestions from my patients about what they would find even more helpful in terms of enjoying a better diet that is really tasty. So in this book you will find even more brilliant ideas, including a chapter devoted to quick dishes you can make in less than 30 minutes (see pages 30–79), giving you lots of ideas for simple, inexpensive weeknight meals as well as for those special meals at the weekend.

There is also a lot of interest in how to maintain the momentum of weight loss and diabetes remission and how to overcome setbacks. As Giancarlo and so many of my patients know, it's all too easy to fall off the wagon and give in to "carb creep". This is why I prefer the term diabetes "remission" to "reversal", because if you drift back to old habits your problems will return. To address this we have included a section on successful behaviour change and its maintenance (see pages 25-29).

Since we wrote the first book, there has been far more acceptance of the low-carb approach. A consensus report by the American Diabetes Association published in 2019 recommends health practitioners counsel people with diabetes "on eating patterns that replace foods high in carbohydrate with foods lower in carbohydrate and higher in fat ,which may improve glycemia (blood sugar), triglycerides, and HDL-C (the helpful cholesterol)".

It's not just about diabetes

When we started our low-carb approach, we were surprised to find significant improvements in blood pressure, weight (particularly reduction in belly fat), liver function and cholesterol and triglyceride levels. Such improvements give the approach a far wider appeal than we ever expected. The initial work was on just 19 patients; six years later, we are finding similar results in hundreds of patients. At the time of writing, I have a research cohort of 267 people who have been low carb for an average of nearly two years. The maximum weight loss is 36kg (about 5½ stone), and the average weight loss is 9.4kg (21 pounds).

I always assumed that older people had a slower metabolism because it slowed with age. Imagine my surprise when we looked at our practice cohort to find that patients aged over 65 lost just as much

> "As my infographics show, it is surprising how much sugar is produced by the digestion of starchy carbs like potatoes, cereals or pasta."

weight as the younger ones! Our oldest low-carb patient so far is 91 years old. Many of my patients choose lifestyle medicine rather than lifelong medication.

Just recently a cardiologist who was writing a paper asked me to examine changes to blood pressure medications for our low-carb patients. I was amazed to find a 20 per cent reduction in prescriptions for these drugs as well as significant improvements in blood pressure. I think this is because carbs cause you to retain salt due to the action of the hormone insulin on the kidneys. On giving up starchy carbs, some people start weeing out the salt their previously sugary diets had caused them to store, with noticeable improvements in blood pressure and ankle swelling. A few weeks ago, a patient with severely swollen ankles lost 5kg (11 pounds) in seven days – a weight loss that must have been mainly water – while marked reductions in his blood pressure meant I was able to reduce his medication. This also explains why it is important that people on prescribed medication should discuss dietary changes with their doctor. Initially, the significant improvements in blood cholesterol and triglyceride we measured were a surprise in view of the butter and other full-fat dairy products we tend to favour. Although it is dietary sugar that turns into triglyceride, a major scientific review in 2018 concluded: "Large randomized controlled trials of at least six months duration with carbohydrate restriction appear superior in improving lipid markers when compared with low-fat diets."

Going low carb: Dr Unwin's quick start

Nutritionist Jenny Phillips expands on going low carb on pages 14–23, but here is my take on low carb in a nutshell. It is centred on the idea of a dramatic reduction in all dietary sources of glucose, so that you will be consuming on average less than 130g (4½oz) of carbs per day. How low carb you go will depend on personal and health circumstances.

• Cut out table sugar completely, if you can. "Cutting back" so often leads to it creeping back at times of stress. People who cut it out are surprised how their tastes and palate change. Now red wine and milk taste surprisingly sweet to me.

• Reduce snacks and treats dramatically. After all, so often they are just more sugar. I opt for almonds, pecans or a square of the darkest chocolate I can enjoy (now 90% cocoa solids, but I started at 70%) and, at the outset, the occasional pure oat biscuit.

• Swap starchy carbs for green veg, unprocessed meat or fish, eggs, nuts and full-fat dairy. It is surprising how much sugar is produced by the digestion of starchy carbs like potatoes, cereals or pasta. A small bowl (150g/5½oz) of boiled potatoes is equivalent to 9 teaspoons of sugar and just one slice of brown bread is like eating 3 teaspoons of sugar.

For the first few weeks it is often easier to keep it simple: easy breakfast choices would be plain, full-fat yogurt with a few berries, or scrambled eggs. If you are hungry, any low-carb meal can become breakfast. Remember: cereals are nearly always very carb-heavy (see below).

Keep other meals simple too. I like the idea of a "mix and match" between protein, green veg and a sauce of your choice. It's how I design nearly all my own meals (see The MealMaker, page 18).

Pick from these protein-rich food: eggs, fish, lamb chops, steak, low-carb sausages (i.e. pure meat, no filler), cheese, chicken legs, sliced ham or beef, canned tuna or salmon. Choose low-carb veg, often, but not always green: broccoli, courgettes, aubergine, cabbage, cauliflower, mushrooms, olives, asparagus, lettuce, rocket and other salad leaves. Add a sauce that fits – pesto, full-fat mayonnaise, melted herb butter, hollandaise, low-carb cheese sauce (or even just cheese grated over hot, green veg), olive oil or similar salad dressing.

Cheese and walnuts or berries and cream could finish off an evening meal. My grandchildren love five or six strawberries or raspberries whisked into double cream with a few drops of vanilla extract. Spooned into a wine glass with a couple of extra chopped berries and a few shavings of dark chocolate, it is good enough for a dinner party.

Drink water, tea or coffee, but avoid too much milk because it contains a teaspoon of sugar in every 100ml (3½fl oz); cream has less sugar in it. The occasional glass of dry wine is allowed too.

Due to the salt that some people lose on a low-carb diet, you may need to add more good-quality sea salt to your meals, particularly at the start.

Finally, I owe so much to my wife Jen. As a clinical health psychologist, she helps people change lifestyle behaviours for the better. In this book, Jen hopes to help you with problems like motivation for change, carb addiction, getting into better habits and learning from setbacks (see pages 25–29). As Giancarlo now realizes only too well, although the benefits of giving up carbs can be substantial, most people suffer the odd setback. As an Italian chef and restaurateur, it was so hard for him to give up pasta and cakes, but he has succeeded – and you can too.

Cutting out sugar and starchy carbs while still enjoying really tasty food, as this book demonstrates, may also bring many other health benefits, including improved liver function, loss of belly fat and healthier blood pressure. But for me, what stands out is the pride people take in being in control of their health – sometimes after years of suffering.

How much sugar in breakfast cereal?

Cereal	GI	Serve size	How does each cereal affect blood glucose compared with one 4g teaspoon of table sugar?
Chocolate rice snaps	77	30g	7.3
Cornflakes	93	30g	8.4
Mini wheats	59	30g	4.4
Shredded wheat	67	30g	4.8
Special K	54	30g	4.0
Bran Flakes	74	30g	3.7
Oat Porridge	63	150ml	4.4

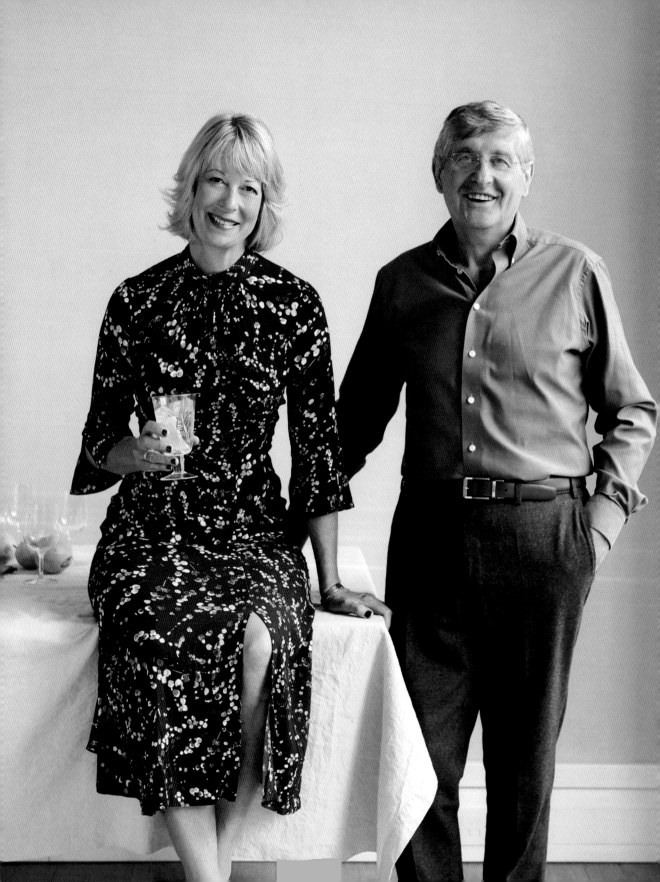

Our
JOURNEY

I fell for Giancarlo, the bright, bouncy, crazy Italian full of energy, fun and impetuous enthusiasm, 23 years ago. I met him when he commissioned me to paint a mural for him in his restaurant. After some months we got together and I entered the world of cooking. We opened restaurants together, and travelled back and forth between the UK and Italy to collect knowledge and recipes. We wrote a book, I learnt to speak Italian, we worked hard, cooked, made a TV series, wrote 12 more cookbooks, had two children and got married.

Around 10 years ago, Giancarlo's enthusiasm for life slowly dwindled. Both of us were overweight and he was always tired. I was testing recipes, writing and bringing up two boys; Giancarlo was working all hours. He would come in after a shift at the restaurant and devour the fruit bowl; two bananas, a whole melon, several oranges. Or he would cook pasta – a huge saucepan full of it. He was so hungry he would sit down with a fork and eat it straight from the pan. If he didn't eat within minutes of arriving home, he was unhappy. While driving he would eat raisins and at each garage stop he would buy biscuits. I began to recognize these mood swings when he was hungry, but I didn't know what they indicated.

His weight gain worsened, particularly around his waist, and he drank bottles of sparkling water to quench his constant thirst. He stopped playing football with the boys because his feet hurt. Even a family walk or trip to the sea saw him sitting it out, not joining in. He developed gout and arthritis. My crazy, fun Italian had become a fat, grumpy man on the sofa, snoring.

One day Giancarlo was driving and his eyesight became blurred. He was able to pull over safely, but it scared him. He felt dizzy and unable to focus. Sensibly, he went straight to the doctor, a private one, because it was a weekend. Within days Giancarlo was told he had type 2 diabetes.

Apparently, he was displaying textbook symptoms of the disease and we were completely unaware. We were sent to see a dietician who advised Giancarlo to cut his portion sizes and reduce his sugar intake. She also told me my waist measurement meant that I could be in danger of becoming pre-diabetic, meaning I would be likely to develop type 2 diabetes. Giancarlo stopped having three sugars in his cappuccino, but otherwise carried on as normal. Looking back, neither of us took it as seriously as we should have done.

Worried about my own weight, IBS and bloated tummy, I gave up gluten. Giancarlo decided to do the same. I felt no different, and yet after just three days he felt amazing. The arthritic swelling in his fingers had visibly reduced and his mind felt clearer. Banning gluten meant that he had to abandon pasta, cakes and biscuits. Luckily, he didn't like most of the gluten-free alternatives. Inadvertently, Giancarlo and I were going "low carb" even though we had never heard of the phrase. We were eating more vegetables, eggs, meat and fish, and less "beige" food. Both of us lost weight and felt better.

To confirm whether Giancarlo was gluten-intolerant, we went to see nutritionist Jenny Phillips. Her tests revealed he reacted very badly to gluten and she advised he should be scrupulous in banning it from his diet for good. It was shocking to hear, but we knew she was right. Knowing Giancarlo was diabetic, she told us to look at the websites www.diabetes.co.uk, www.lowcarbprogram.com and www.dietdoctor.com.

This was a turning point for us. Living and eating low carb for us both and gluten-free for Giancarlo was the way forward and we both lost weight easily. At the time, we were writing *Around the World in Salads,* and this way of eating a full rainbow of foods chimed fully with our new lifestyle. Within 18 months Giancarlo had lost 3 stone and put his diabetes into remission.

Both of us are passionate in wanting to share our story and spread the word that type 2 diabetes should be taken seriously, but at the same time reinforcing that you can help yourself back to health and away from this condition through diet, not drugs. We have loved creating recipes that satiate and are easy to produce.

Giancarlo feels great and I have a new slim husband, full of energy and fun once more. I have lost the weight that bothered me for years and kept it off. Our teenage boys have gradually become more low carb and feel better for it. We have never insisted, but they have seen the transformation in their dad and don't want to suffer in the way he has.

Low carb is not a crash diet – it has been our way of life for six years. The low-carb lifestyle is about eating fresh, natural foods that don't overload your bloodstream with glucose from sugar and starch. We are low carb, not no-carb. There are so many people recovering from eating disorders that I would hate to think we are suggesting another form of over-controlled eating. I feel strongly that we are giving people information as to what happens to food in your body and then, armed with that knowledge, people must make their own choices. We all react differently to food, hence the CarbScale on page 15.

We are not carbphobes either. If I want a bowl of pasta or a pizza, I will have it and thoroughly enjoy every mouthful. I cannot resist the warm focaccia at our restaurants, but I limit bread to a couple of times a month and I won't feel guilty about it. Giancarlo lets himself have a treat once a week, otherwise he would feel too restricted. Dr Unwin completely avoids sugar and bread, as he doesn't want to be tempted back into eating too many biscuits or a whole loaf. Find what works for you.

Our top tips for going low-carb

● Ask yourself if you really are hungry. Sometimes thirst can seem like hunger, so drink plenty of water and often the feeling goes away.
● Just because your watch says it is 8am, 1pm or 7pm, it doesn't mean it is time to eat. Eating just twice a day helps us keep trim. It's amazing how your appetite drops when you are low-carb. I always used to wake up hungry; now I have coffee and cream, and don't eat until lunchtime. If I've had a big lunch, I'll often skip dinner, which means I can stay in a fasted state for longer.

"Quality, quantity, movement."
Giancarlo's mantra

● Don't eat between meals. There is no need, so be strict with yourselves. That slight hunger pang is ok, you won't faint. Your body will have to use some of the stored fat for energy. Let it do its job and don't overfeed it.
● Don't eat quickly. It takes a while for your body to recognize you have had enough to eat.
● Eat like the Japanese; they eat a variety of foods slowly and mindfully from small bowls. Once you have eaten some pickled vegetables, slurped your miso soup, picked up every grain of rice and cut up fish or meat with chopsticks, you are not really hungry. They have an expression: "Hara Hachi Bu", meaning eat until you are 80 per cent full and stop.
● The French start their meals with a salad and the Italians have antipasti; both take the edge off hunger so that you don't then devour a huge main course.
● The Mediterraneans don't drink without food. Have a few olives with a drink, then you won't miss the bread.
● Visualize the ingredients that you are eating on a plate, and if it resembles a pile of flour, poor-quality fats, colourings and flavourings, E numbers and unpronounceable chemicals, don't eat it.
● Just try to cook. Don't worry if you fail every now and again; everyone does – yes, even Gordon, Jamie and Delia! Enjoy cooking and experimenting. Bring in your family and ask them to taste and help.
● Eat more vegetables and enjoy their huge variety of flavours and textures. Fall in love with cabbage, cauliflower, pumpkin and swede; we have. They make perfect substitutes for potatoes, bread, pasta and rice.
● Low carb doesn't have to be expensive. We have included plenty of thrifty options using canned fish, lentils, chicken, frozen spinach, meat and fish, and lots of recipes with eggs and vegetables.
● Use every excuse to move more. Sitting down is unhealthy. I know, I spend most of my life writing, but I stand up frequently, tilt my screen up and do squats while I read and lunges while on the phone. I probably look barmy, but I like my new shape and don't want it to change.

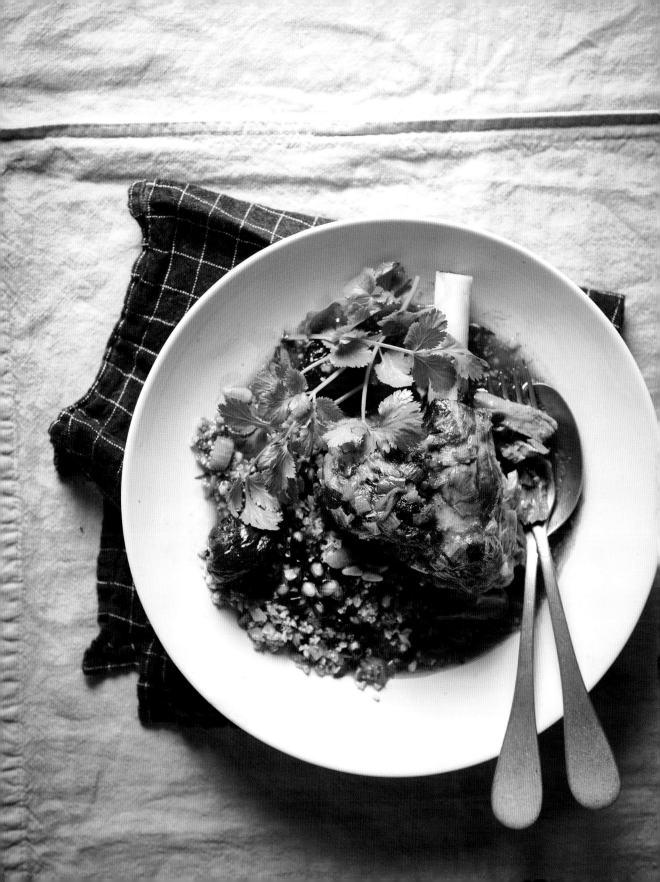

The POWER of FOOD

Jenny Phillips, nutritional therapist

Working as a qualified nutritionist, I have the pleasure of helping people to use diet and lifestyle to improve their overall health and wellbeing. This is how I met the Caldesis and together we were able to put Giancarlo's type 2 diabetes into remission by changing his diet.

In *The Diabetes Weight-loss Cookbook* we discussed just how powerful the low-carb approach is in achieving a healthy weight and also improving blood sugar regulation – the key goal of diabetes management. But it can do so much more, as Dr Unwin has already described (see pages 4–9). This is because your blood sugar is managed by the hormone insulin, which pushes the glucose into cells either to make energy or to store energy as glycogen or fat, which is why obesity and diabetes often go hand in hand. Long before glucose levels start to rise above normal levels, it is likely that insulin levels will also be running high, and the cells become less responsive to it. This is known as insulin resistance.

There are many health conditions that involve insulin resistance. These include:

- type 2 diabetes
- obesity
- cardiovascular disease
- cancer
- dementia
- hormonal imbalance, such as Polycystic Ovary Syndrome (PCOS)

The good news is that we know how to improve insulin sensitivity, which is the opposite of insulin resistance, and that is by limiting our intake of sugar and the refined or starchy carbs because these rapidly break down into sugar during digestion. This strategy is the prime focus of this book: a low-carb approach to eating.

A further issue that may resolve with a low-carb diet is indigestion. This is a very common problem. Symptoms include acid reflux, bloating, gas or erratic bowel habits. This eating plan may help improve your digestion because:

- You eat a lot of vegetables, which are a good source of soluble fibre.
- We exclude refined grains, such as wheat, which can be difficult to digest.
- We encourage you to have a go at making sauerkraut (page 107) to give a boost to your gut bacteria. Your plan also includes prebiotics – food for the good bugs – such as onions, leeks, garlic, asparagus and psyllium (a type of fibre that can be used in baking).

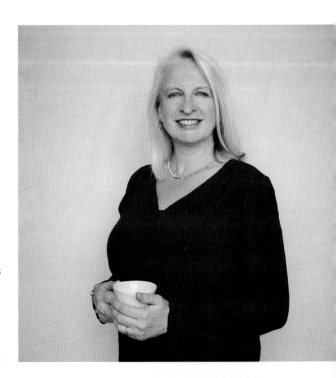

The CarbScale

STRICT LOW CARB	MODERATE LOW CARB	LIBERAL LOW CARB
You have type 2 diabetes or are looking to lose weight	You are trying to maintain weight or lose a few pounds, but are otherwise healthy	You are fit and active, and need to keep calories up
Carbs around 50g (1¾oz) a day	Carbs 75–100g (2–¾3½oz) a day	Carbs up to 130g (4½oz) a day
Everyone can enjoy: **Protein** – meat, fish, eggs, nuts, seeds, dairy | **Non-starchy vegetables** – mostly vegetables that grow above ground | **Good fats** – olive oil, butter, dairy, coconut oil and fats found in meat or fish | **Treats** – see the recipes in chapter 5 (pages 164–189), dark chocolate		
Keep carb intake low to optimize blood sugar levels and lose weight; occasionally add fruit or pulses combined within a meal to add variety	Add some fruit, starchy veg, pulses and the occasional off-plan meal, maybe with pasta or soda bread	Also consider adding oats or modest portions of rice, pasta or quinoa, depending on your energy requirements
Try to avoid: Pizza, pasta, pies, biscuits, shop-bought cakes, muffins, doughnuts, sweets, milk chocolate, commercial bread, cereals, porridge, crisps, pretzels, sugar-sweetened drinks like cola, refined vegetable oils, margarines, etc. Always check the ingredients list (see page 19).		

Making low carb work for you

Low-carb eating is a delicious and sustainable way to achieve your health goals. Following our guidelines ensures that you won't go hungry or experience dips in energy. Here are our three top tips to get you started:

1. Eat real food, generously!

Low-carb eating encourages using fresh ingredients, but it doesn't have to mean spending hours in the kitchen! In essence, you combine protein with lots of non-starchy vegetables, good-quality fats and some carbohydrates, depending on your own tolerance. We call this the CarbScale, which reflects the fact that low carb has a broad appeal but there can be individual nuances, depending on your own metabolism and energy needs.

It's really important that your meals are substantial and satisfying. The combination of good fats and protein helps to keep you feeling fuller for longer so that you don't feel the need to eat or snack as often. These two macronutrients are also essential, which means they must be included in your diet for optimal health. This may surprise you, especially if you've been following a low-fat diet, but here is why fats are essential:

● Every cell of your body has a membrane that is a bi-lipid layer – meaning, made up of two layers of fat. This gives the cell structure and controls what enters and leaves the cell – a very important job.

● Your brain is 60 per cent fat, and your nervous system is protected by a fatty layer called the myelin sheath (rather like the insulation around an electrical wire).

● All of your sex hormones and the stress hormone cortisol are derived from cholesterol, an important fat-based molecule.

● You can use fat to make energy – it contains more than twice the calories per gram of carbs.

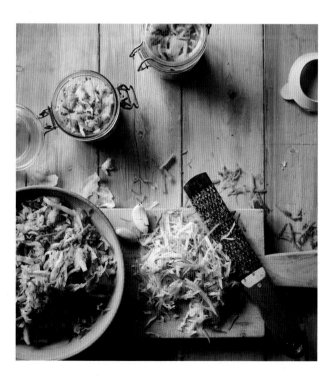

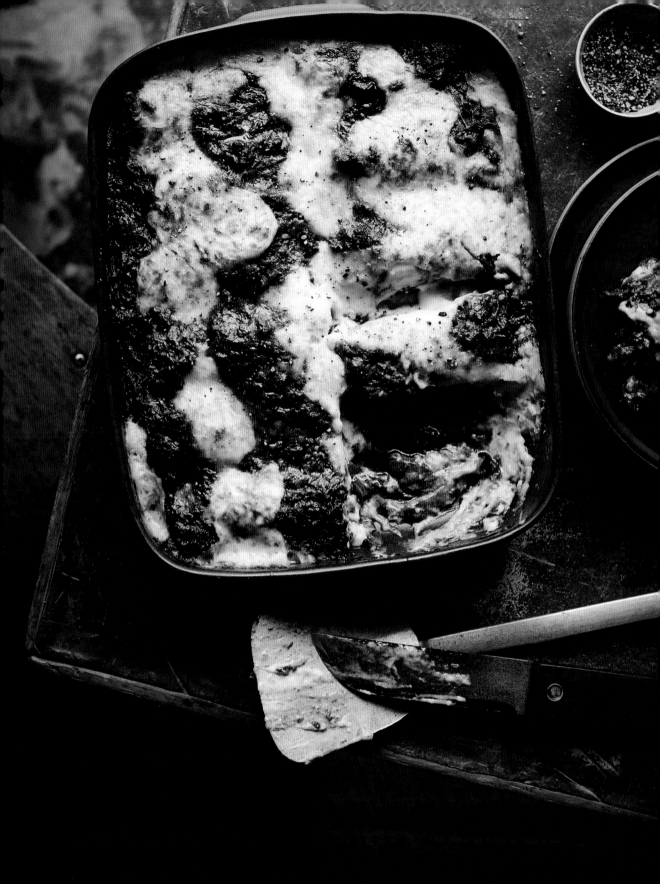

- Only fatty foods contain the fat-soluble vitamins:
  - retinol, the active form of vitamin A, which supports good vision and immune health
  - vitamin D, for bone and immune health
  - vitamin E, a powerful antioxidant, that helps to protect your cells
  - vitamin K_2, which is involved in calcium metabolism and hence bone and heart health

You may already have a sense that protein is an important macronutrient. It is used to build and repair tissues, build muscle, bones and skin and also to make enzymes, hormones and other important chemical messengers including:

- adrenaline – a stress hormone
- dopamine – the "reward and motivation" hormone
- insulin – regulates blood sugar
- serotonin – the "happy" hormone
- thyroxine – controls your metabolic rate

The third macronutrient, carbohydrate, is not essential. However, it is a source of calories and fibre for good digestion. Vegetables, which contain carbs, are also a fantastic source of vitamins, minerals and antioxidants. Try to eat slow-release carbs, depending on where you are on the CarbScale.

2. Take a break – the benefits of Intermittent Fasting (IF)

IF can be as simple as eating three good meals per day with nothing in between. Snacking is a modern invention and the current advice of "eat little and often" may not be helpful for many people (although exceptions could be if you are very unwell or need to gain or maintain weight).

When I first followed a programme requiring three meals and no snacks, with only water between meals, I was not happy! I always planned for several healthy snacks and believed the dogma of eating little and often. I was shocked to find out this simply wasn't true. Instead, IF was truly liberating.

I now coach most of my clients to follow three good meals a day with about 5 hours in between, which gives an "eating window" of 10–11 hours and an overnight fasting period of 13–14 hours.

Quite simply, when you fast, provided you have low insulin levels, you switch into burning fat stores.

As Dr Unwin mentions (see page 6), your body is like the engine of a hybrid car – running beautifully on either fat or glucose.

This is liberating because eating less frequently saves both time and money. It is convenient, as you don't constantly need to be searching for food. The other brilliant benefit of IF is that you can regulate your weight easily without reducing your metabolic rate. Once you become "fat adapted" (using fat as energy), it becomes easy to reduce the number of mealtimes further to reduce your calorie intake, without feeling hungry. We all now frequently skip breakfast, and on one day a week I eat one meal.

In contrast, even the smallest low-calorie snack can cause fat-burning to grind to a halt. Low-calorie foods are almost always low fat, which means that they are mostly carbs and hence they increase insulin levels. Unfortunately, this prevents your body from being able to access fat stores; instead, it faces a calorie deficit that can, over time, reduce your metabolic rate. In a study of people following a combination of calorie restriction and vigorous physical exercise, significant weight loss was achieved but at the expense of the Resting Metabolic Rate (the number of calories required to maintain life). This reduced by more than 700 calories a day and means that when normal eating is resumed rapid weight gain becomes almost inevitable.

3. Know your sugar equivalents

For some time now, the media have made us aware of the amount of sugar in popular foods and drinks. But a big breakthrough in managing diabetes came when Dr Unwin established the sugar equivalents tables now endorsed by NICE. For the first time, both medical experts and the public alike could see instantly the issue with many of the refined and starchy carbs that are a mainstay of our diets.

Starchy foods are made up of strings of glucose molecules, which are broken down by your digestion. These foods break down very quickly, releasing glucose into the bloodstream, which drives up insulin levels. If you are eating starchy foods "little and often", then you are constantly challenging your body's ability to control your blood sugar and keeping insulin levels high, which can have a range of potential health issues over the long term (see page 14). Look at the tables on page 7 to see just how "sugary" many popular foods are.

Becoming low-carb savvy

Once you understand the strong scientific basis for low-carb eating, the next step is how to do it. Later in this section (see page 23) we provide a meal plan which you can follow, or you can simply swap some new recipes into your current favourite choices.

We are conscious that sometimes you just need a quick and easy way to put meals on the table. Hence, we designed a shortcut that we have called the MealMaker (see right). Simply take one portion of protein, two or three portions of vegetables, top with a tasty dressing to add calories and enjoy! These can be cooked or cold (otherwise known as a salad!). Here are some tips to help you get started.

How much can I eat?

Overall, the calories you require depend on your own size, metabolism and activity levels. Experiment to find the amount of food that suits you.

To maintain calories eating low carb you need to increase your intake of good fats. Daily protein needs are a minimum of 0.8g per kilo of body weight, which is 56g (2oz) for someone weighing almost 70kg (11 stones).

Assuming an average calorie intake of 2,000kcal per day, your split of macronutrients could look like the illustrations opposite.

To increase your fat intake:
- enjoy fatty cuts of meat and oily fish
- cook using olive oil, butter, coconut oil or animal fats like dripping
- use olive or speciality oils for sauces and dressings
- enjoy dairy products
- include avocado and olives in salads
- use nuts and seeds liberally

If you have weight to lose, then consider combining low carb with intermittent fasting (IF – see page 17) – the goal is to mobilize body stores of fat while reducing overall calorie intake. In this way you become a "fat burner" rather than a "fat storer".

Reading labels

It really pays to get a handle on how many carbs you are eating; this need not be forever, as you soon learn where the dangers lie. However, it always pays to read food packet labels, as you can never be sure of what's inside.

The MealMaker
Great low-carb meals made simple

PROTEIN	VEG	SAUCE OR DRESSING
Meat	Non-starchy:	Parsley Salsa Verde
Chicken	eat generously	(page 38)
Turkey	Asparagus	Quick Italian Tomato
Beef	Aubergine	Sauce (page 50)
Pork	Avocado	Mushroom Cream
Lamb	Broccoli	Sauce (page 58)
Game	Brussel sprouts	Bacon Tomato & Chilli
	Cabbage	Sauce (page 47)
Fish	Cauliflower	Pecorini Cheese
Salmon	Celeriac	Sauce (page 55)
Cod	Celery	Tahini Dressing
Mackerel	Courgette	(page 52)
Sea bass	Cucumber	Chimichurri Sauce
Tuna	Fennel	(page 60)
Other fish	Green beans	Shogayaki Sauce
	Kale	(page 64)
Vegetarian	Leeks	Ponzu Sauce (page 71)
Eggs	Lettuce	Lemon Crème Fraîche
Cheese	Mushrooms	(page 74)
Beans	Okra	Jar dressings
Lentils	Olives	(page 79):
Nuts & seeds	Onions	*Creamy Vinaigrette,*
	Peas	*Lemon & honey,*
	Peppers	*Balsamic & lemon,*
	Pumpkin	*Vinaigrette*
	Rocket	*One-minute*
	Spinach	*Mayonnaise (page 78)*
	Tomato	*Lemon Yogurt*
	Watercress	*Dressing (page 89)*
		Tomato Relish
	Starchy: eat	(page 123)
	according to	Coriander & Mint Raita
	the CarbScale	(page 131)
	(see page 15)	
	Beetroot	
	Butternut squash	
	Carrots	
	Parsnip	
	Swede	
	Sweetcorn	
	Turnip	

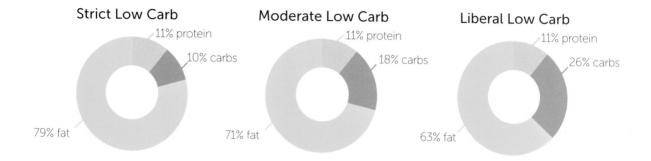

Strict Low Carb
11% protein
10% carbs
79% fat

Moderate Low Carb
11% protein
18% carbs
71% fat

Liberal Low Carb
11% protein
26% carbs
63% fat

First, look at the ingredients and shop for products including ingredients you recognize. Ultra-processed products are linked with worse health outcomes; these contain additives not commonly used in the kitchen such as flavour enhancers, thickeners and emulsifiers. Try reading out a long list of unfamiliar ingredients on a packet and ask someone what the contents might be. Sometimes it is very hard to identify a food without the brand name!

Next, look at the nutrient information. This can be expressed per 100g, enabling comparison between different products, or by portion size or both. Beware of portion size, as these may be underplayed to appeal to calorie counters. A twin pack that you intend to eat may have the nutrient information for just half the pack. Most cereal packets suggest a serving size of just 30g (1oz), yet most people pour two to three times this amount into a bowl.

Here is an example of a nutrition label:

	Per 100g	Per portion
Energy	456kcal	192kcal
Fat	17.2g	7.2g
Carbohydrate	64.5g	27.1g
Of which sugars	28.3g	11.9g
Fibre	5.6g	2.4g
Protein	8.1g	3.4g

This product, which is a healthy-looking oat bar, is 64 per cent carbs, which is very high. As a rough rule of thumb, look for 20 per cent or less. Per portion, this product clocks up 27g (over 1oz) of carbs!

"Of which sugars" is a subgroup of total carbs – it includes both added and natural sugars, found, for example, in milk or fruits. A low-sugar product

means less than 5 per cent of the total calories. If sugar features early in the ingredients list, then you know it has a lot of added sugar.

Fibre is the indigestible part of the food and is usually, but not always, a subgroup of carbs.

Net carbs are a quick calculation to estimate the amount of carbs that are available to the body; simply subtract fibre from the total carbs. In this case, the portion of net carbs is 27.1–2.4g = 24.7g (almost 1oz). That is still high!

You are looking to optimize protein and good fat. Per portion here is 3.4g protein and 7.2g fat, which is low compared with the amount of carbs. Calories are a less important consideration, as your goal is to manage insulin release through controlling carb intake. If I'm grabbing a meal on the go, I often shop for the highest calorie and lowest carb option, as this is more satisfying and helps me to eat less often.

Of course, when you cook at home, the nutrient info is not readily available, which is why we have included it with every recipe here. Alternatively, you may like to track carbs using something like Carbs & Cals (available as a book or app) or other fitness apps (such as MyFitnessPal).

Alcohol

"What can I drink?" is a really common question. Try to keep drinking to social occasions – a glass or two sat on the sofa will likely see your intake escalate.

Spirits, red wine or dry white wine are good options. Beer and cider are very carby. The issue with spirits is which mixer to use. Either use low-calorie mixers or top up with soda water and a slice of lemon or lime. I add a teaspoon of elderflower cordial to gin with lots of soda and ice, which keeps sugar intake low (but not zero). Katie has included lower carb drinks ideas on pages 186–188.

It's also important to be aware that regular drinking is not good for long-term health. NHS guidelines advise that you consume no more than 14 units per week, which equates to 5 glasses of wine (200ml/7fl oz) or 3 large spirit measures (50ml/2fl oz). Alcohol is also a source of empty calories (meaning it contains no nutrients), which won't help you to achieve your weight-loss goals.

Sweeteners

As you transition away from sugar you might find it helpful to use sweeteners. However, this could delay resetting your taste buds and therefore your habits. Even better, try to abstain and within two weeks your cravings for the sweet stuff should decrease.

We do have some desserts for you (see chapter 5), and typically these use just a tiny amount of dates as a natural sugar. We also use a very small amount of honey in some dressings. In all instances, this has a minimal effect on the total carb level of the dish.

Exercise

While "you can't outrun a bad diet", exercise can help in your quest to improve your health or lose weight. Exercise improves insulin sensitivity, and releases endorphins, which make you feel happy. A short walk after dinner is a good place to start.

There are two community-based exercise programmes worthy of a mention. Parkrun is supported by many GP surgeries and offers weekly 5km running (or walking) events all over the world. They are free and open to all. Another is GoodGym, which combines a "good deeds" programme with exercise. Once signed up, you are matched with a small local project, such as moving some furniture for an elderly lady. You run there as a team, help out, run back and clock up community goodwill!

Before you begin

Just to reiterate two points that Dr Unwin has already made (see pages 4–9), if you are on medication for diabetes or blood pressure, then do speak with your health professional before making changes to your diet. This is so that they can monitor you and adjust medication if required.

Also, be aware that lower insulin levels can result in a loss of sodium, so add good-quality salt to your meals to compensate. If you feel light-headed in the first few days, then add a teaspoon of salt to water.

Exercise improves insulin sensitivity and releases endorphins, which make you feel happy.

Low-carb out & about

This book contains recipes for when you're on the go (see pages 80–107) to help if you are out for the day. Sometimes you may prefer to eat out, so below is some advice on how to choose the best low-carb options, whether it's grab and go, coffee shops, restaurants or takeaways.

Grab & go

The good news is that combining intermittent fasting with higher-fat, low-carb eating means you are not constantly hunting for food, but there might be times when you need to shop on the go. Always check the ingredients and choose against higher-starch ingredients like bread, rice and pasta. Some supermarkets are becoming increasingly low-carb savvy, and generally it is easy to grab portions of meat or fish that can be teamed with salad, or

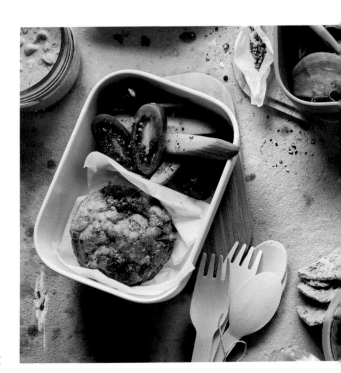

choose cheese, nuts, olives, etc. Remember to scan the nutrient info (see page 19).

Coffee shops

Who doesn't love meeting friends for a coffee? Unfortunately, coffee shops are often a carb haven and so you need to employ some self-control. An Americano is a better choice than cappuccino or latte because milk contains a significant amount of carbs as lactose – just 125ml (4fl oz) milk is equivalent to 1 teaspoon of sugar. Some chains can offer cream instead of milk, which tastes more luxurious (helping keep you off the muffins!), feels more satisfying and is zero carb. And of course, don't add syrups or sugar – you're sweet enough!

Consider keeping some low-carb snacks handy – Katie takes walnuts and 90% dark chocolate to have with coffee to keep her off the carrot cake! I cycle regularly and take a small tub of nuts and apple wedges with cinnamon in my saddle bag.

Restaurants

Low-carb eating out need not be difficult, and many people find it easier than when following a calorie-controlled diet. Here are some considerations for you, and tips for eating in pubs and Italian, Indian and Chinese or Thai restaurants.

- If you don't know the restaurant, try looking at the menu online beforehand so that you know what's on offer.
- Focus on protein and veg, if necessary, swapping out the carbs for another vegetable or salad.
- A burger is fine; just ditch the bun.
- Say no to the bread basket. If it sits on the table, it might be tempting.
- Add olive oil generously to salads to bump up calories and satiety.
- Consider a coffee with cream in place of a dessert.

Pubs: You may need to go more upmarket to find a pub that offers veg, although all should have salad options. Avoid chips, sandwiches and deep-fried (ie battered or breaded) foods.

Italian: Usually offer a wide choice of meat or fish, often including liver, which is a superfood in terms of the amount of nutrients it contains. Many vegetarian options are quite carby (pizza, pasta),

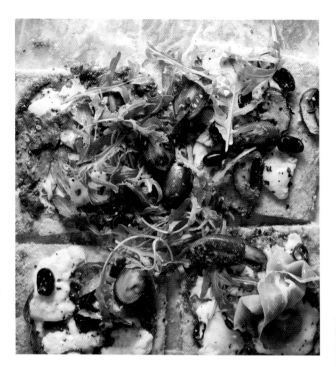

although dairy may be an option (mozzarella, etc). Or ask for pasta sauces served over veg. The Caldesis offer a range of low-carb options in their restaurants – ragù served over shredded cabbage tossed in butter or roasted veg are delicious favourites. You could also ask for this elsewhere, as most restaurants should be able to rustle this up quite easily.

Indian: Go easy on or even ditch the poppadums, rice, chapatis and naan; instead, fill up on veggie sides such as spinach, mushrooms and chickpeas. Indian restaurants offer great variety for both meat eaters and vegetarians, as they widely use different pulses such as dal (lentils) and paneer. Consider ordering meat without the sauces because these can be very sweet. You may like to ask if your meal could be cooked in ghee (clarified butter) rather than refined commercial oils (aka bad fats).

Chinese/Thai: Go careful with the rice and also the noodles, which can cause big swings in blood sugar levels. Beware battered or deep-fried foods, and those served with sweet sauces (even black bean sauce has sugar in it!) Some Chinese restaurants offer lettuce wraps with crispy duck, for instance. Choose meat or fish dishes with vegetables, either stir-fried or in a satay (peanut) sauce. Thai foods often have sauces made with coconut milk, which is a good choice.

Takeaways

Calling out for food is such a simple and convenient thing to do, but it can also mean relying on meals that are often carb-heavy and cooked in refined commercial oils. Take a look at the chapter on Fakeaways (see pages 108–135) to see if you could make something simple and similar at home. If you do order a takeaway, follow the guidelines for restaurants (see page 21) as best you can.

High days & Holidays

How to manage feasting times

There are three times of the year in particular when weight can typically increase – around the Christmas, Easter and the summer holidays. In addition, there may be personal celebrations where you find yourself with the potential to go "off piste" from your eating plan. Jen Unwin discusses the emotional side of eating on pages 25–29 and shares ideas to get you back on track.

Here are some practical tips to help you through the holiday season.

1 **Check in with yourself:** Try to establish a regular routine for weighing yourself, maybe once a week. Once the scales start to move, you can take action more quickly and limit the damage.

2 **Buddy up:** Sharing a weigh-in with a friend can be motivating and you can help each other by sharing goals and ideas. It also introduces a healthy competitive element, provided you are both happy with this.

3 **Drink a glass of water before you eat:** Studies show this can help to reduce the calories consumed when we eat freely, and may help you to control your appetite. Water is also a better choice than diet sodas with a meal too, as the latter may stimulate appetite. Obviously watch your alcohol intake (even wine, which is low carb, can have nearly 200kcals per glass) and avoid sugary drinks.

4 **Take a low-carb dish to share:** The buffet table can be a nightmare, as it tends to be groaning with beige foods – pastries, sandwiches, crisps, pizza and so forth. This is even more of an issue if you like these foods and are trying to avoid them. So, take something you enjoy and spread the low-carb joy.

5 **Use feast and famine:** Intermittent Fasting (IF – see page 17) is your secret weapon and helps you to reduce your overall calorie intake during the day. You could fast after an indulgent lunch, or the next morning after a lovely dinner. Don't force mealtimes when you don't need to. Often, we eat out of habit or to be social rather than because we really need food.

6 **Explain to your host if you are cutting carbs for health reasons:** Most often, it is completely fine to tweak menus to accommodate you – just focus on protein and vegetables; dessert could simply be fruit and cream, or cheese.

7 **Plan ahead if possible:** I frequently travel with low-carb bread (see page 101), nuts, apples and dark chocolate.

8 **Be active:** While it is often the case that you tend to eat more when on holidays, you may also have a bit more time to exercise. Encourage friends or family members to join you for a walk, or indulge in your favourite exercise.

"You could fast after an indulgent lunch, or the next morning after a lovely dinner. Don't force mealtimes when you don't need to. Often, we eat out of habit or to be social rather than because we really need food."

Weekly meal plan

We hope you are inspired by the wonderful recipes in this book and want to encourage you to add them to your own meal repertoire. This meal plan highlights some of our favourites and shows how they can come together over the course of a week.

Don't worry if you just want to pick out a few recipes to start with, alongside some of your own favourite dishes. You also may want some meals to be a bit simpler, in which case you could use the

MealMaker (see page 18), which is a shorthand way of planning a protein, vegetables and tasty sauce combination with the minimum of fuss.

You may also like to cook extra portions and save for the next day. For example, Kathryn's Super Simple Stir-fry (page 58) could double up as a lunch. Your choice of crackers (page 85) or low-carb bread (page 101) can also cover several days so that you don't have to cook from scratch each and every time.

	BREAKFAST *Add tomatoes, avocado, mushrooms or low-carb bread (page 107)*	LUNCH *Add low carb crackers (page 85), bread (page 101) or salad*	DINNER *Add lots of vegetables!*
Monday	Feta & Red Pepper Omelette (page 36)	Spiced Red Lentil Soup (page 54)	Kathryn's Super-simple Stir-fry (page 56)
Tuesday	Simple Scrambled Eggs (page 40)	Broccoli, Ginger & Coconut Soup (page 48)	Pezzi with Bacon, Tomato & Chilli Sauce (page 47)
Wednesday	Greek yogurt & berries	Green Bean "Linguine" with Tuna Puttanesca (page 51)	Toad in the Hole & Onion Gravy (page 150)
Thursday	Magic Muffin (page 96)	Smoked Mackerel Fishcakes (page 74)	Sausage Ragù & Cauli-Rice Pilaf (page 67)
Friday	Low-carb Rolls (page 101) with bacon & avocado	Salmon, Lemon & Parsley Pâté (page 84)	Chicken Tikka Masala (page 128)
Saturday	Stuffed Omelette with Creamy Mushrooms (page 36)	Quick Fried Paprika Spiced Chicken (page 89)	Mexican Sea Bass with Pico do Gallo Salsa (page 76)
Sunday	Goat's Cheese, Mushroom & Thyme Scrambled Eggs (page 41)	Layered Tuna & Pepper Frittata (page 93)	The Burger & Sesame Bun with Tomato Relish (pages 123–124)

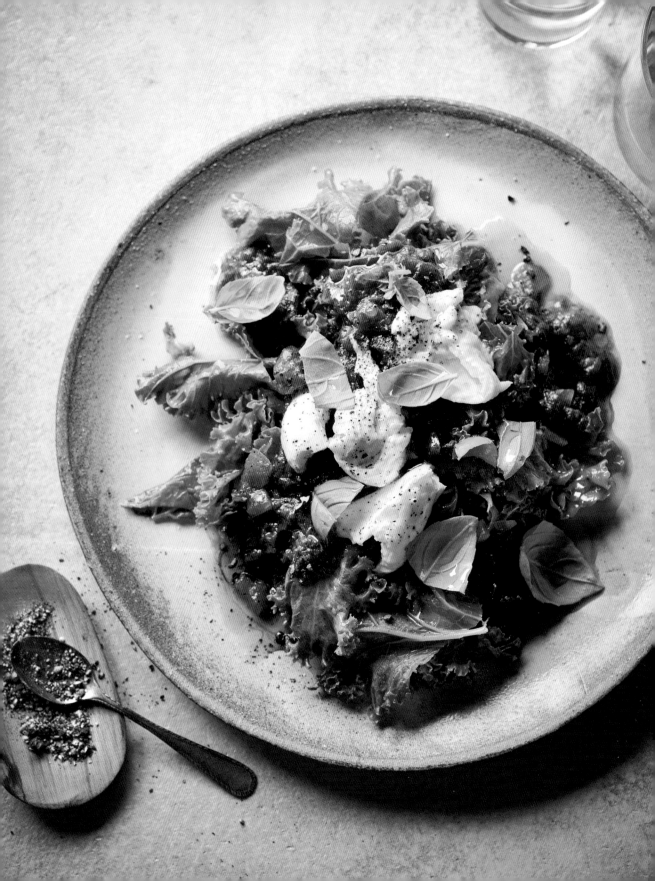

Tips for long-term success
Jen Unwin, NHS psychologist

For six years now I have been helping my husband David to run low-carb groups in his GP practice. As a clinical health psychologist, I'm fascinated by the links between mind and body and how we can use them to help people improve their lives. I think nearly everyone who has tried reducing sugar and refined carbohydrate (bread, pasta, rice, baked goods, etc) in their diet will tell you of the rapid benefits they notice in their overall health and wellbeing. Weight loss, more energy and improved digestion and sleep are common after the first week or so. However, despite these great early results, many people genuinely struggle to make a permanent lifestyle change to low-carb eating. It is so worth persevering; at times you may experience setbacks and feel the switch is too difficult, but here I can offer psychological insights to help you maintain, sustain and enhance your new healthy approach to nutrition. The keys to success are: understanding your motivation, and the role of food addiction for some people, using the power of habits and developing a mindset based on learning what's right for you in the long term.

Motivation

I've developed a super-easy way for you to think about motivation and changing your behaviour. David and I use it in the low-carb groups we organize in his practice. We also teach this model to other health professionals and use it on ourselves and in our family. We call it GRIN to help you remember the four stages, and also because evidence shows that people with this goal-focused mindset are happier. Happy people enjoy a whole range of benefits, including better health and wellbeing, and even living longer! Let's explore each stage so that you can think how it might apply to you in adopting a low-carb lifestyle or making other changes in your life.

Goals

This first stage is the most important and is the bedrock of motivation. Always start with what you are hoping for: what does success look like to you? Tell someone else about it or write it down perhaps. Try to make your goals as clear as possible. People often say to us, "I want to lose weight" or

"I would like my knees to stop hurting" or, in chef Giancarlo's case, "I would like to walk better". How about your goal? What are you hoping will be better if you improve your diet? Then we always take it a step further and ask: "What difference would that make to your life?" People have a think and then say something like "I could play with my grandchildren" or "I could enjoy my retirement with my wife", or, again in Giancarlo's case, "I can carry on running my restaurant and be around for my boys and Katie".

In my clinical practice as a psychologist, I find that the more people imagine a better future, the more likely they are to make it happen.

> Despite these great early results, many people genuinely struggle to make a permanent lifestyle change to low-carb eating.

- Can you imagine a better future?
- What would be better about it?
- Don't worry too much about "how" at the outset!

Resources

The next stage is listing all the things that are already on your side in achieving your goal. First, what are your personal strengths and characteristics that will help you? Don't be coy! For example, I'm naturally a very organized person, so I bring that to managing my weight and taking regular exercise. Are you determined, or a team player, or brave or energetic? How might you use your best traits to achieve your goal? If you are at a loss, try the free strengths test at www.authentichappiness.sas.upenn.edu.

Second, who might you enlist to help you? A spouse, sibling, co-worker, friend or online community, such as www.diabetes.co.uk or www.dietdoctor.com. It's encouraging to make changes with others and there are many inspiring people around who have similar goals.

Last, and importantly, what is already working and going well? We tend to forget this. For example, are there times when you manage to eat more healthily? Maybe at work? Are you already exercising? Are you someone who prepares food from scratch and enjoys cooking?

Scaling is another psychological way to think about this: if your goal is represented as 10/10, then on a scale of one to ten, where are you already and why? Perhaps you have given up mid-afternoon biscuits or sugar in your tea. Keep doing the things that are already working.

Increments

This leads nicely into the next stage. Say you are already at 3/10, as you go to the gym twice a week and eat well at lunchtimes at work because you take a salad you prepared at home. Then the next increment would be to get to 4 and to decide what that would represent. What would tell you that you were now 4/10? Maybe pre-planning your evening meals as well as lunches. Maybe cutting out pasta or rice with dinner. Your next steps will be unique to you and, of course, must feel achievable.

Noticing

Finally, it's really important to pay attention to what works and to any small positive changes. So many of us dwell on negative symptoms like pain or anxiety. Try actively looking out for positive improvements instead. Supposing you had pre-planned your

dinners for a week, or given up sugary breakfast cereals. What difference did it make to you? How did you feel? Would you say that you feel a bit nearer to your goal? Why?

Also included in "noticing" is asking; what are the best forms of feedback for you to plot your progress? In the practice, we plot graphs of weight, waist circumference or relevant blood tests (see below). Some of you will have seen on Twitter that David @lowcarbGP sometimes features one of his patients as "graph of the week". Feedback is a vital part of behaviour change and is essential to long-term maintenance. What might you measure that fits with your goal to help with this?

Reframing "failure"

As I said at the beginning, many of us will experience setbacks as part of our low-carb journey. I recall visiting Giancarlo and noticing he had gained weight again and didn't look as well, but then a few months later he looked better than ever – he was back on track. In clinical practice, it's common to see people (often after a holiday or Christmas) who are annoyed to have "slipped back". Disappointment can so easily become a negative spiral, causing you to think it's hopeless. We encourage people to reframe this as a learning opportunity. After all, don't most of

Sustaining weight loss
(weight in kg)

Regular weight measurements are good for feedback and to keep track of progress.

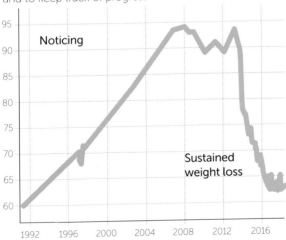

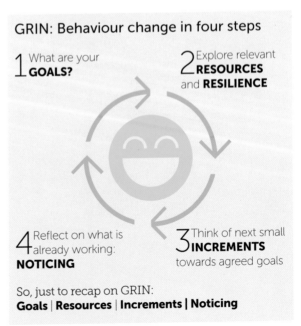

GRIN: Behaviour change in four steps

1 What are your **GOALS?**

2 Explore relevant **RESOURCES** and **RESILIENCE**

3 Think of next small **INCREMENTS** towards agreed goals

4 Reflect on what is already working: **NOTICING**

So, just to recap on GRIN:
Goals | Resources | Increments | Noticing

us learn some of our best lessons from mistakes?

What were the mistakes you made? Be specific. So what would you do differently next time? I remember over one Christmas I gained a stone and a half! That was a disaster I never wanted to repeat. So, for the next year, we planned a low-carb Christmas, in advance.

Look at the graph below showing one of our client's weight over several years. Can you see how he is learning from mistakes and every time his weight loss is improving?

Habits v. willpower

I mentioned in our first book that habits and long-term lifestyle change are vastly superior, over time, than willpower. Even for those of us with considerable determination, willpower can and does wane, especially when we are tired or stressed. Then we berate ourselves. Far better to work out what works well for you and make small but permanent changes to your everyday routine. Habits built up like this take very little mental energy to maintain. For instance, most of us are in the habit of brushing our teeth without a thought in the mornings; it takes no real discipline at all. Here's a personal example: a few years ago I gave up breakfasts as routine and now it seems very unusual to have it (say on holiday,

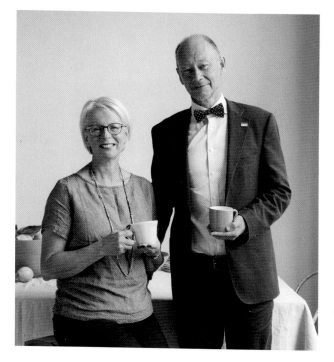

perhaps). Likewise, we always decline the bread basket in restaurants and now that seems normal. It's true to say that even after seven years living low carb, we are still refining how we do it and what works best. When we learn something new online or at a conference, we have a go and see whether we feel better or if it's easier. If so, we carry on; if not, we go back a step. A lifelong attention to what keeps you at your best will ensure that you are focused on wellbeing and making small improvements.

All that may sound a little self-indulgent. But most of us are needed by our families and colleagues, and if we can bring our best selves to every occasion, then that is good for everyone. We are all unique. There is no magic one-size-fits-all diet. For example, I can't moderate how much I eat very easily, so I have learnt to fast intermittently (see page 17) and avoid certain foods, such as peanut butter, so that I can maintain a healthy weight. David doesn't tolerate cheese well, so he avoids that but still enjoys cream and butter.

Learning from mistakes (weight in kg)

If you fall off the wagon be honest about the circumstances and come up with a plan to do something different next time.

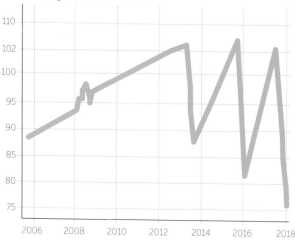

Sugar and dental health

James Goolnik BDS, MSc, dentist and founder of the charity Rewards Project

Dental disease is one of the first indicators that your diet is a problem. Your mouth is a barometer of what else is happening in your body. If you are struggling with your blood sugar levels, your dentist often knows about it before your doctor.

I want to focus on two common aspects of dental disease – tooth decay and gum disease. Tooth decay is the most common bacterial infection in the world. It happens when the food in your diet is eaten by the bacteria in your mouth and the by-product is acid. This acid dissolves your teeth – they decay! Every person has a different mix of bacteria in their mouth and some are more aggressive than others, which is why some people can eat lots of sugar and never have a cavity and others need a filling every six months. The best thing you can do is to cut down on feeding these bacteria the food they love. Sugar is their favourite, but they can also live off carbohydrates. The fastest route to tooth decay is to eat a mix of sugar and carbs, such as doughnuts. These sticky foods hide from your toothbrush in hard-to-reach places and can rot your teeth in as little as three months.

Research has shown that eating these foods at mealtimes is slightly better than having them as snacks, but why not give your teeth a break and just avoid them completely? Dental decay can be entirely prevented: don't feed the bacteria and never have another filling again!

A second major problem is gum disease, which is worse in diabetic patients. Gum disease is an inflammation of the structures that hold in your teeth. It starts with slight swelling and redness around your gums (gingivitis), and they bleed when you brush. Please do not ignore this bleeding. Make an appointment immediately with your dentist or hygienist and get them to help you. If left, this inflammation spreads down your gums causing them to peel away from your teeth, then the bacteria eats away at your bone (periodontitis), causing your teeth to loosen and eventually drop out! Eating a healthy low-carb diet reduces the inflammation in your entire body, including your mouth. You cannot enjoy these delicious recipes with no teeth!

Sugar addiction

A number of people have significant lifelong struggles with overeating sugary and carb-heavy foods, particularly if they are combined with fat – toast and butter, pizza, crisps, doughnuts and chocolate, for example. Sugar and fat do not occur naturally together in real foods and the combination has powerful effects on our brain chemistry. The food industry relies on us finding it hard to moderate our consumption of such hyperpalatable foods (see opposite). Also, sugar is available everywhere in our environment (at home, work, in garages, cinemas,

> Regular and good-quality sleep may help balance dopamine levels and there is some evidence that meditation can also raise levels naturally.

even fitness centres and hospital waiting areas, and, of course, in restaurants and supermarkets). We certainly didn't evolve to cope with this daily onslaught. Not everyone is truly addicted to sugar, but a proportion of people are. It is likely that genetics, childhood experiences and emotional factors all play a strong role. Most people struggle to cut down on sugar and carbs, but in some ways doing so is even more important for those of us with an addictive relationship to food. You wouldn't advise an alcoholic to drink in moderation.

Here are some signs that your relationship to carb-heavy foods may be addictive in nature:

● Eating more than you intended and finding it hard to stop eating certain foods.
● Wanting to cut down on certain foods but being unable to.
● Spending a lot of time thinking about and obtaining certain foods.
● Strong cravings and urges to eat certain foods.
● Continuing to overeat even if it is causing strain in relationships.

- Giving up important social events, hobbies or job opportunities because of weight/overeating.
- Eating certain foods over and over again even when you know they are doing you harm physically and/or psychologically.
- Needing more and more of certain foods to get the same effect.
- Experiencing "withdrawal" symptoms when you abstain from carbs/sugar that are relieved by consumption.

If you recognize these patterns in yourself, then a low-carb diet may help you to escape the addiction trap. We have found that people who gave up carbohydrate in their diet were, in time, freed from cravings. However, if you think there may be addtional emotional issues underlying your use of food for mental comfort, then consider a 12-step programme such as Overeaters Anonymous, or find a psychologist who specializes in eating issues or consult your own doctor for advice.

How can food be addictive? There are a number of mechanisms that have been suggested. The first is the hyperpalatability of manufactured foods combining sugar, fat and salt that can hijack our appetites. Eat real, wholefoods and avoid processed foods in packets. Second, when we eat sugar or carbs insulin is released. In the presence of insulin, an amino acid, tryptophan, can more easily cross into the brain where it helps to produce and be made into serotonin, the major feel-good hormone regulating mood. However, over time, if this process is repeated, tryptophan and hence serotonin will be depleted, leading to low mood and anxiety. A third mechanism is that sugary foods stimulate the reward centre in the brain, releasing dopamine, which is linked to reward and motivation. This means we are likely to repeat behaviours that lead to its release. Over time, the repeated consumption of sugar reduces the dopamine receptors in the brain. Hence, we feel the need for increased consumption to get the same results and sometimes withdrawal from other activities.

Once we understand how carbohydrate can hijack our brain chemistry, we can decide to maximize serotonin and dopamine in other ways to support kicking sugar out for good. There are ways to boost serotonin naturally, for example by taking regular exercise (especially outdoors, as daylight is also important) and eating foods rich in tryptophan (turkey, chicken, eggs, cheese, beef, salmon, tuna, nuts – all low carb!). In terms of increasing dopamine, the advice is to eat plenty of beef, eggs and turkey, which contain tyrosine that the body converts into dopamine. Iron, vitamin B6, niacin and folate are needed to produce dopamine and these too are found in meat. Regular and good-quality sleep may help balance dopamine levels, and there is some evidence that meditation can also raise levels naturally. Sunlight is important in regulating dopamine, explaining the winter blues.

Modern life has not only led to a rise in metabolic diseases but also in mental health problems. The answers don't lie in more tablets but in lifestyles that redress some of the imbalances. Nutrition is an important bedrock of good health as Jenny Phillips explains (see pages 14–23). Link nutrition with exercise, quality sleep and good social relationships and you will be unstoppable!

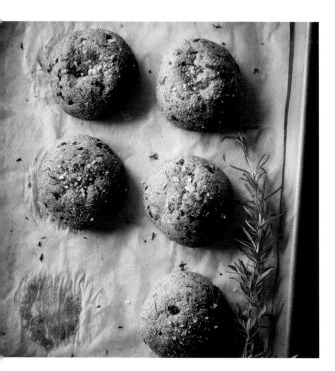

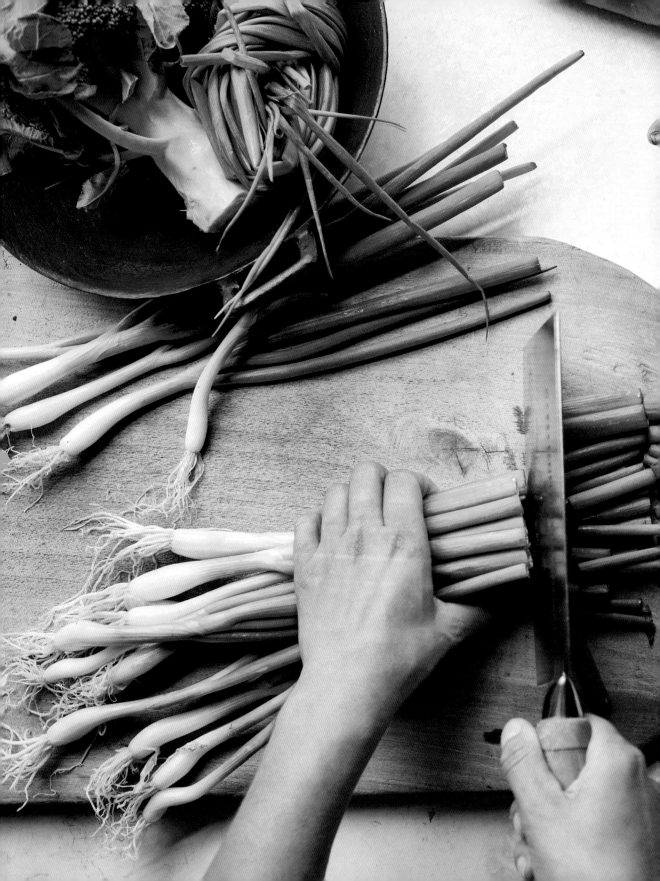

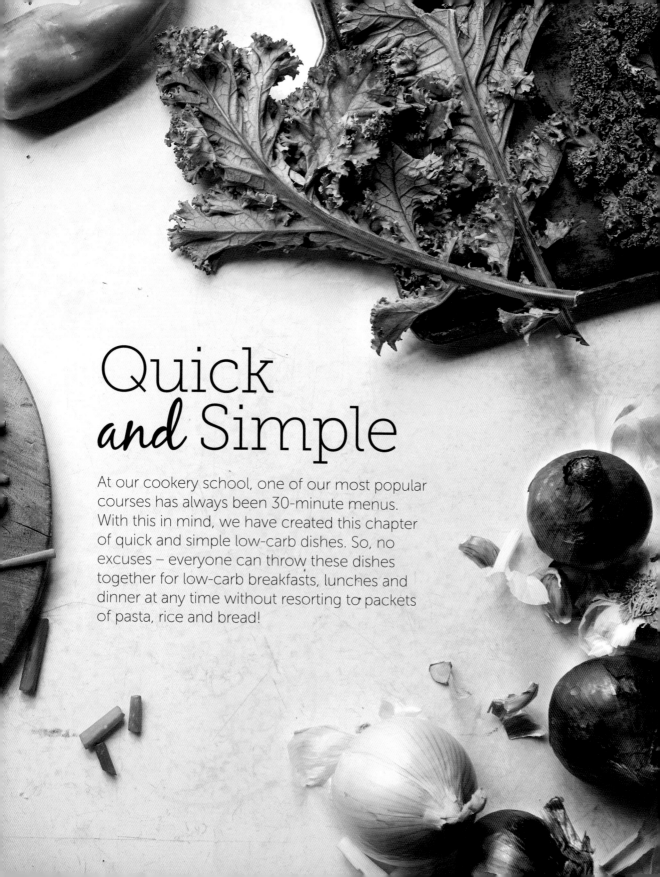

Quick *and* Simple

At our cookery school, one of our most popular courses has always been 30-minute menus. With this in mind, we have created this chapter of quick and simple low-carb dishes. So, no excuses – everyone can throw these dishes together for low-carb breakfasts, lunches and dinner at any time without resorting to packets of pasta, rice and bread!

Artichoke, Mushroom, Pepper & Spring Onion Antipasti Salad

This Italian fry-up is ideal as a starter, light lunch or supper. Artichokes in water are cheaper than the ones in oil and by adding your own oil you can be sure you are using olive oil rather than seed oil. However, do use jars of artichokes in oil if that is all you have. Don't be tempted to use balsamic glaze as it is contains sugar. Canned palm hearts, fresh asparagus and wedges of red onion are good added to the pan and are handy substitutes for any ingredient that you might not have in or dislike. To eke out the meal, add a sliced avocado, a sliced mozzarella ball, cured meat or the Pissaladière (page 154) or the Rosemary & Olive Rolls on page 101 to the party. The oil from the pan tastes amazing after it has absorbed the flavours of the vegetables, so we use it to make the dressing.

Heat the oil in a frying pan or griddle pan and fry the spring onions, mushrooms and pepper (lay them skin side down on their backs) until just starting to brown, which will take about 5 minutes over a high-ish heat. Season them in the pan.

Meanwhile, halve the artichoke hearts lengthways and season with salt and pepper. Remove the onions, mushrooms and pepper as soon as they are browned and set aside on a warm plate. Add the artichoke hearts to the pan, cut side down, and fry them until lightly browned. Keep the pan and cooking juices for the dressing.

Transfer the fried artichokes to the warm plate. Now arrange the salad leaves on a wooden board or large plate and put the warm vegetables next to them (not on top or they will wilt).

For the dressing, pour the balsamic vinegar and the oil into the pan with the juices and heat for 2 minutes over a high heat to reduce the vinegar. Season to taste, then pour over the salad just before you serve with the Parmesan shavings over the top.

SERVES 2 (OR 4 AS A STARTER)

4 tablespoons extra virgin olive oil
4 spring onions or 1 onion, cut into 8 wedges
250g (9oz) chestnut mushrooms, halved
1 red pepper, cut into 8 lengths
1 x 390g (13½oz) can artichoke hearts in water (240g/8½oz drained weight), drained
1 small head of soft lettuce, leaves separated, or a bag of mixed leaves
25g (1oz) Parmesan shavings, made with a vegetable peeler
salt and freshly ground black pepper

For the dressing
1 tablespoon balsamic vinegar
2 tablespoons extra virgin olive oil

Per serving 9.7g carbs, 4.4g fibre, 5.8g protein, 33g fat, 366kcal

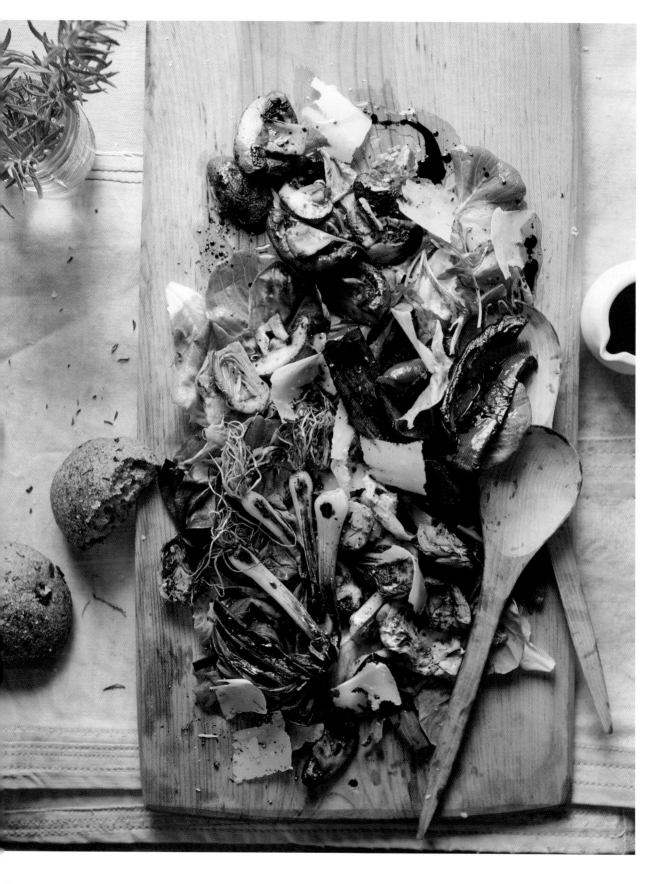

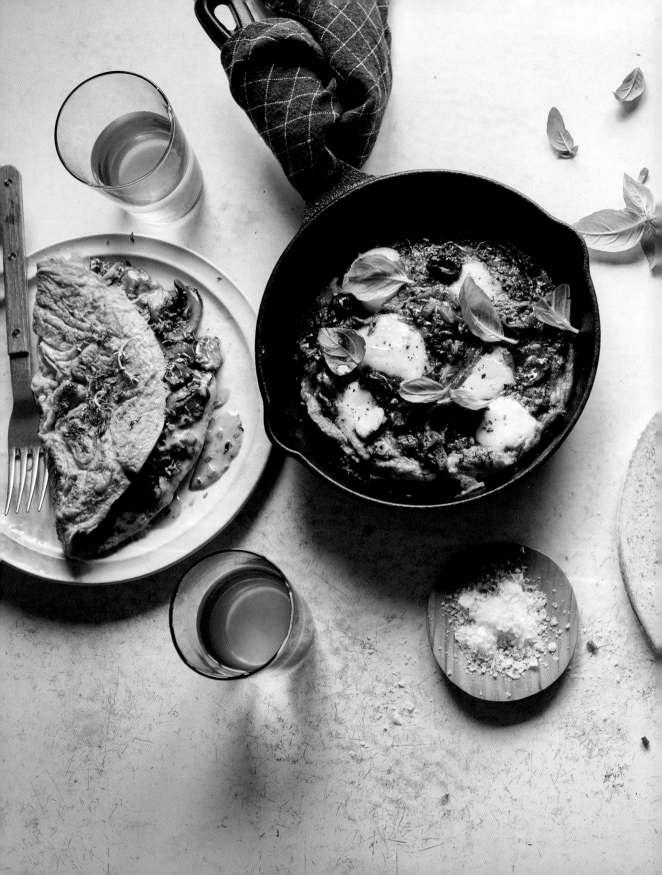

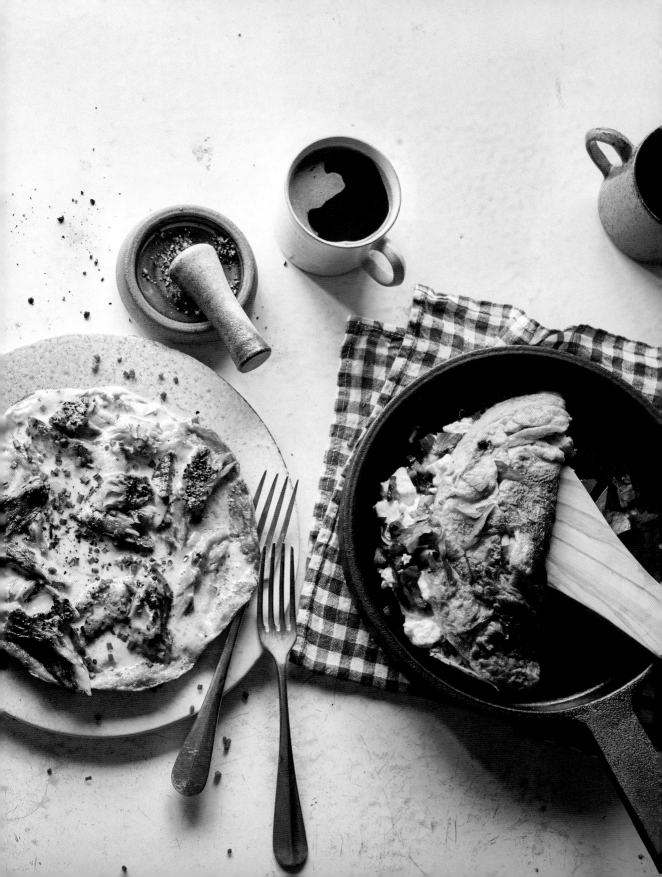

4 ways with... OMELETTES

Omelettes tend to get forgotten in our house for a year or so, then resurrected in a different form and we wonder how on earth we did without them. Omelettes are the perfect low-carb meal, ready in 5–10 minutes, and lend themselves perfectly to using up leftovers. I have used 3 medium eggs, which I find enough for two, but do bump up to 4 if you are especially hungry or have the whole 3-egg omelette to yourself if you are only eating twice a day.

Feta & Red Pepper Omelette

Enjoy these folded straight from the pan, or finished under the grill or puffed up and proud from a hot oven.

Make sure you have a warm plate ready and everything you need to hand to work quickly. Use a fork to beat the eggs in a small bowl with the seasoning until well combined (chopped herbs can be added now, if using). Heat a non-stick frying pan over a medium heat. Add the oil and butter to the pan and swirl it around as the butter melts to coat the base of the pan. Increase the heat to high and when the butter starts to foam, add the eggs.

Use a spatula to move the eggs around for about a minute, criss-crossing the pan to get the runny eggs to the bottom. When the outer edges become opaque, run the spatula around the rim of the pan to loosen it. Shake the pan to make sure the omelette can slide.

When the bottom is almost set and cooked to your liking, add your filling ingredients to half the omelette. Use your spatula to flip the uncovered half over to encase the filling. Slide the omelette onto the warm plate to serve.

SERVES 2
For the basic omelette
3 eggs
1 teaspoon extra virgin olive oil
10g (¼oz) butter
¼ teaspoon fine salt and freshly ground black pepper

For the filling
fresh herb leaves, such as parsley or coriander, roughly chopped (optional)
¼ red pepper, finely diced or coarsely grated
3 tablespoons crumbled feta

Per serving 1.3g carbs, 1.8g fibre, 17g protein, 16g fat, 216kcal

Stuffed Omelette with Creamy Mushrooms

This dish makes an impressive breakfast or quick lunch. Serve it with a few cut and seasoned tomatoes, and a little parsley, basil or thyme.

Preheat the oven to 200°C/180°C fan/400°F/gas mark 6.

Follow the instructions above using an ovenproof pan. When the eggs are almost set on the base, remove the pan from the heat. Spread the creamy mushrooms over half the omelette. Use your spatula to flip the uncovered half over to encase the filling. Transfer the pan to the oven. Cook until the egg is set; about 5 minutes should do it. Remove the pan from the oven and slide the omelette onto the warm plate. Scatter with the herbs.

SERVES 2
1 quantity of Basic Omelette (above)
1 quantity of Mushroom Cream Sauce (page 58), hot or at room temperature
1 tablespoon finely chopped herbs, such as parsley, coriander, chives

Per serving 5.6g carbs, 3g fibre, 15g protein, 55g fat, 627kcal

Pizza Omelette

I have to admit I was cynical about this concept, as I thought the egg flavour would be dominant, but actually it is completely delicious and has become a family favourite.

Preheat the grill to hot. Follow the instructions for Feta & Red Pepper Omelette (see opposite) using a pan that is suitable to transfer to the grill. When the eggs are almost set on the base, remove the pan from the heat. Dollop on the tomato sauce and spread it gently with a spatula just to the edges of the omelette. Evenly scatter over the oregano and olives, distribute the salami, if using, and tear over the mozzarella.

Put the pan under the hot grill for 2–3 minutes or until the mozzarella has melted and the edge of the omelette has risen and browned. Using oven gloves, remove the pan from the grill and slide the pizza omelette onto the warm plate. Scatter over the basil and enjoy.

SERVES 2

1 quantity of Basic Omelette (opposite)
5 tablespoons Quick Italian Tomato Sauce (page 50) or passata with seasoning
½ teaspoon dried oregano
8 black or green olives, pitted
6 slices of salami, or spicy sausage or 6 anchovy fillets (optional)
75g (2¾oz) mozzarella, drained
fresh basil leaves

Per serving 2.7g carbs, 2.1g fibre, 22g protein, 35g fat, 422kcal

Arnold Bennett-style Omelette

Invented in 1929 by a chef at the Savoy Hotel in London for the novelist Arnold Bennett, this omelette is usually so heavy with cream and cheese you can do nothing but have a lie-down after eating it – scarcely write a novel. In this simplified version, we use ready-cooked peppered mackerel and spoonfuls of crème fraîche to lighten the result and speed things up.

Preheat the grill to hot. Follow the instructions for the Feta & Red Pepper Omelette (opposite), using a pan that is suitable to transfer to the grill. When the eggs are almost set on the base, remove the pan from the heat.

Use your hands to break the fillets of fish into bite-size pieces and scatter these and the cheese evenly over the omelette. Dollop over the crème fraîche and put the pan under the grill for 2–3 minutes or until the eggs are puffy and golden brown. Using oven gloves, remove the pan from the grill and slide the omelette onto the warm plate. Serve scattered with the parsley and some freshly ground black pepper.

SERVES 2

1 quantity of Basic Omelette (opposite)
2 x 70g (2½oz) smoked peppered mackerel fillets
25g (1oz) Parmesan, Grana Padano or Cheddar, finely grated, plus 10g (¼oz) for the top
4 tablespoons full-fat crème fraîche
1 tablespoon finely chopped parsley or chives
freshly ground black pepper

Per serving 1.8g carbs, 1.4g fibre, 32g protein, 63g fat, 705kcal

Pumpkin, Pepper & Halloumi Traybake with Lemon & Parsley Salsa Verde

Warm up the oven, raid the fridge and get supper on the table within 30 minutes with this fast, colourful and delicious traybake. Any vegetables will work here including broccoli, aubergine, green beans or cauliflower. Go for a variety of brightly coloured vegetables, add the chickpeas for crunch and the cheese for satiety. Try to find the small capers in brine or salt, which taste better than the large ones; a jar keeps in the fridge for months. Use the remaining chickpeas in the Spinach Falafel on page 86 or freeze them, along with any extra halloumi or sliced pumpkin.

Preheat the oven to 240°C/220°C fan/475°F/gas mark 9.

Put the vegetables, herbs and garlic into a large mixing bowl with the oil, salt and pepper and toss through. Spread in a single layer on a baking tray and roast for 20 minutes.

Remove the tray from the oven and add the chickpeas, tossing them into the vegetables and spreading them out in a single layer. Scatter the halloumi over the top and return the tray to the oven for 10 minutes or until the cheese has browned and the vegetables are cooked through and lightly charred.

To make the dressing, pile up the parsley, capers, garlic and lemon zest on a board and chop them finely together. Put this into a bowl and stir in the lemon juice, oil and oregano. Add salt and pepper to taste and set aside.

Serve the traybake on the tray with the dressing drizzled over the top or pile on two plates with the dressing in a jug on the side.

SERVES 2

200g (7oz) pumpkin or butternut squash, cut into pieces about 1cm (½in) thick
1 red onion, sliced or 6 spring onions
1 red or yellow pepper, sliced
1 courgette, cut diagonally into long slices
1 tablespoon chopped thyme leaves or a few whole sprigs
2 garlic cloves, unpeeled and lightly crushed
3 tablespoons extra virgin olive oil
120g (4¼oz) cooked or canned, drained chickpeas
110g (3¾oz) halloumi, cut into fingers or cubes about 2cm (¾in) wide
salt and freshly ground black pepper

For the dressing
a large handful of parsley
1 heaped teaspoon small capers, rinsed
1 small garlic clove
finely grated zest and juice of ½ lemon
4 tablespoons extra virgin olive oil
½ teaspoon dried oregano

Per serving (using pumpkin)
25g carbs, 8.7g fibre, 22g protein, 53g fat, 677kcal
Per serving (using butternut squash) 31g carbs, 10g fibre, 22g protein, 53g fat, 705kcal

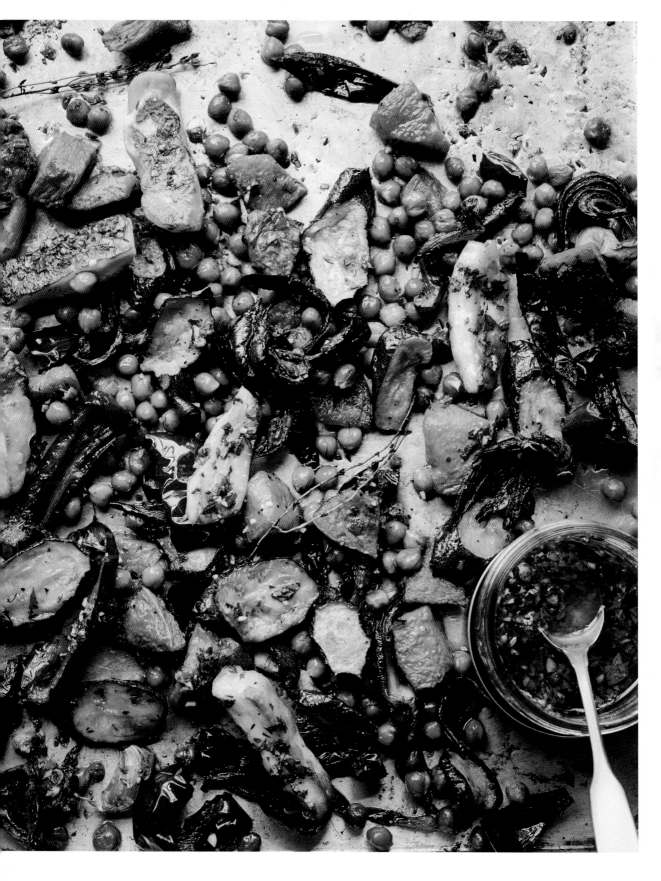

4 ways with... SCRAMBLED EGGS

Basic scrambled eggs – eat as they are, or with the simple addition of tomatoes and herbs, smoked salmon or bacon and mushrooms. But scrambled eggs shouldn't be consigned to breakfast only – in Kolkata I was served them spiced up and punchy for a light dinner. In Turkey they were part of a brunch and were so good that Giancarlo and I went into the kitchen and asked the chef for the recipe. In turn, he asked us to show him how to make fresh ravioli, so it seemed a fair swap.

For Simple Scrambled Eggs

Beat together the eggs, cream and seasoning in a mixing bowl with a fork.

Melt the butter over a low heat in a non-stick large frying pan until it starts to foam. Pour in the egg mixture and stir continuously as it begins to set. Move the runny eggs and solid areas together until it is cooked to your liking. Remove from the heat and serve straight away.

SERVES 2
4 eggs
2 tablespoons double cream or crème fraîche
½ teaspoon salt
a few generous twists of black pepper
25g (1oz) butter, ghee, coconut or extra virgin olive oil

Per serving 0.5g carbs, 1.8g fibre, 15g protein, 29g fat, 327kcal

Menamen – Turkish Scrambled Eggs

This is simple and lovely on its own or, to spice it up, add a little fresh or dried chilli. It is also good with sliced avocado or crumbled feta on top.

Beat the egg mixture together as above.

Fry the onions, garlic, green pepper and ginger together in the butter (above) for about 5 minutes over a low heat or until the onions have softened. Then add the tomatoes and heat through. Pour in the beaten egg mixture and gently stir through. Scatter over the parsley to finish.

SERVES 2
1 quantity of Simple Scrambled Eggs (above)
3 spring onions or ½ white onion, finely chopped
1 small garlic clove (optional)
½ green pepper, thinly sliced
a small knob of ginger, peeled and grated (optional)
200g (7oz) fresh or canned tomatoes, finely chopped
a few sprigs of parsley, finely chopped

Per serving 5.1g carbs, 3.3g fibre, 16g protein, 29g fat, 362kcal

Indian Eggs

This spicy Indian version is so delicious and takes scrambled eggs to the next level. Eat on their own or with a side salad or the Turmeric Cauli-Rice on page 66.

Beat the egg mixture together as opposite.

Fry the onions, tomatoes, chilli, garlic and ginger using the butter (opposite) in a large non-stick frying pan over a medium heat for 2–3 minutes until just starting to soften.

Add the curry powder to the beaten egg mixture. Pour the egg mixture into the pan and stir through as opposite. Dollop on the yogurt and scatter over the coriander. Serve straight away.

SERVES 2

1 quantity of Simple Scrambled Eggs (opposite)
2 fat spring onions or 1 shallot or ½ pepper, finely chopped
6 cherry tomatoes, halved
¼–½ green chilli, finely chopped, or a pinch of chilli powder
1 fat clove garlic, finely chopped
a small knob of ginger, peeled and finely chopped
1 teaspoon curry powder
50g (1¾oz) Greek yogurt
a small handful of coriander leaves, stalks finely chopped

Per serving 2.3g carbs, 2.3g fibre, 24g protein, 39g fat, 456kcal

Goat's Cheese, Mushroom & Thyme Scrambled Eggs

Use any mushrooms for these, such as chestnut or button. If you don't like goat's cheese, substitute it for another kind.

Beat the egg mixture together as opposite.

Fry the mushrooms in the oil with the thyme over a high heat for about 7 minutes until soft.

Reduce the heat to low, pour the beaten egg mixture into the pan and stir through as above. Dollop on the goat's cheese. Serve immediately

SERVES 2

1 quantity of Simple Scrambled Eggs (opposite)
125g (4½oz) mushrooms, sliced
3 tablespoons extra virgin olive oil
a few sprigs of thyme
75g (2¾oz) soft goat's cheese

Per serving 2.3g carbs, 2.3g fibre, 24g protein, 39g fat, 456kcal

Stuffed Hispi Cabbage with Ricotta on Quick Italian Tomato Sauce

This very simple recipe for stuffed cabbage rolls is very easy to put together and cooks quickly. The leaves are soft enough to simply roast and don't need any pre-cooking. The ricotta filling is lovely as it is or add a little more flavour with a couple of slices Parma ham, four slices of cooked and chopped smoky bacon or a couple of tablespoons of finely chopped sun-dried tomatoes and a little thyme.

Preheat the oven to 200°C/180°C fan/400°F/gas mark 6. Put the tomato sauce in the base of an ovenproof dish measuring about 24 x 20cm (9½ x 8in).

Make the stuffing by mixing the nutmeg, seasoning, ricotta and grated cheese together in a bowl. Add any additional chopped fillings at this point and stir them through.

Spoon half the stuffing into the centre of each cabbage leaf and spread it out with the back of the spoon. If you are adding Parma ham, lay a slice on now. Roll up each leaf in a spiral.

Turn the leaf over so that the spine faces upwards and make several shallow cuts through the roll all the way along its length. Each cut should only be about 5mm (¼in) deep. This allows the heat to penetrate through the roll easily and cook the stem. If the stem is particularly large, you can cut some of the end away at an angle. Each leaf is different, so it's up to you.

Lay the cabbage spirals on the tomato sauce, drizzle over the olive oil and give each one a pinch of salt and a twist of black pepper.

Bake for 20 minutes or until the cabbage is just soft and starting to collapse.

MAKES 2 ROLLS

½ quantity of Quick Italian Tomato Sauce (page 50)
¼ teaspoon freshly grated nutmeg
100g (3½oz) ricotta
25g (1oz) Grana Padano, finely grated
2 large leaves from a hispi, sweetheart or pointed cabbage
2 tablespoons extra virgin olive oil
salt and freshly ground black pepper

Optional:

4 rashers cooked bacon, roughly chopped
2 heaped tablespoons finely chopped sun-dried tomatoes
2 sprigs of thyme, leaves only
2 slices of Parma ham

Per serving 11g carbs, 2.3g fibre, 23g protein, 52g fat, 619kcal

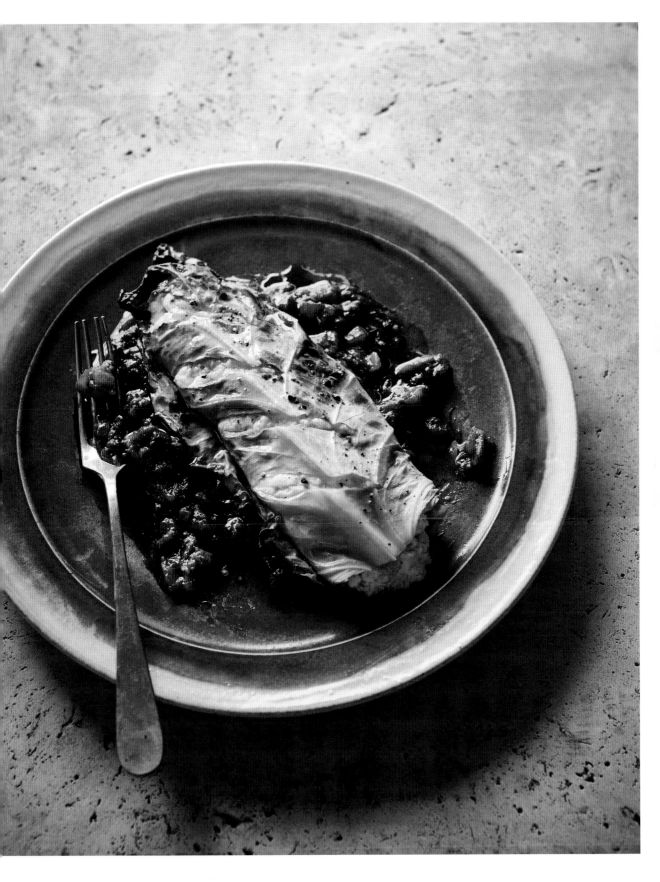

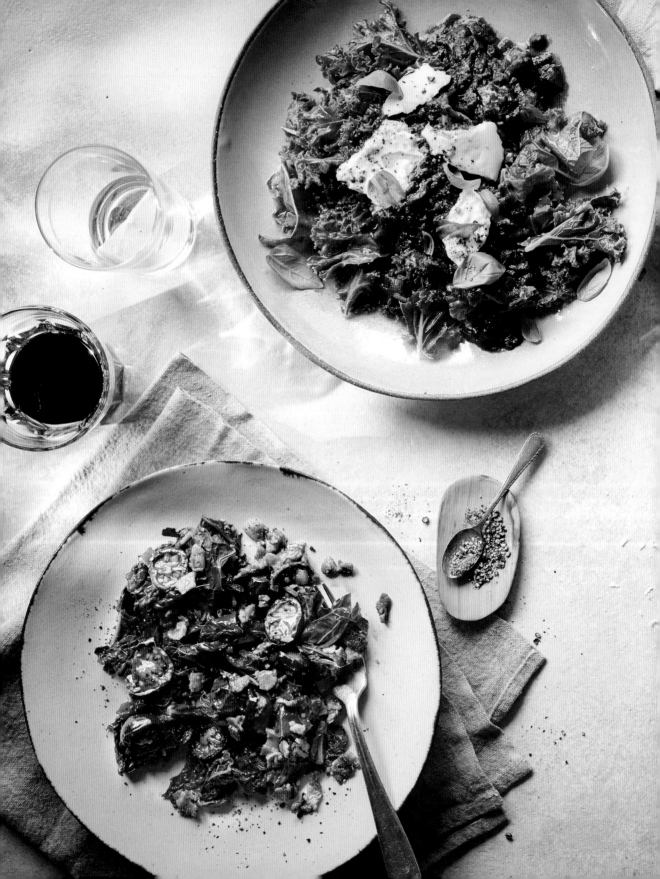

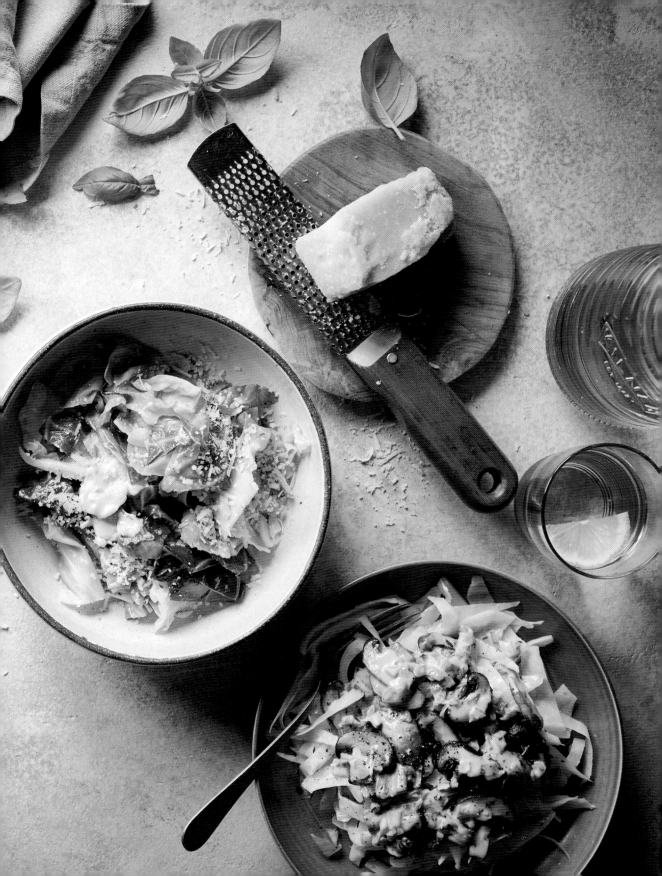

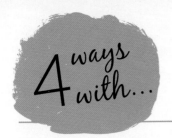

4 ways with... PEZZI

"Pezzi" in Italian means "pieces" and it has become our word for cabbage in our household when we use it instead of pasta since we've gone low-carb. Pezzi are quick to prepare and incredibly versatile. All the cabbage family will work as pezzi but have different cooking times. White cabbage, being firmer, will need to cook for a couple of minutes longer than either Savoy or kale to transform it into soft, tender pieces.

Hispi Pezzi with Butter & Cheese

This makes a simple side dish to sausages, roast meats or a cheese main course. It is also good with a couple of poached eggs on top.

Remove any very tough stems, damaged leaves or hard core from the cabbage. Tear or cut the leaves into pezzi about 5–7cm (2–2¾in) across or roll them up and cut into tagliatelle-style ribbons. Put it into a microwave bowl with the salted butter, water and salt and pepper. Cover with a plate and microwave on full power for 5–7 minutes, stirring halfway through.

Alternatively, put the cabbage into a medium saucepan with the butter, water and seasoning and cover with a lid. Cook over a medium heat for 5–15 minutes or until it is almost transparent and tender; this will depend upon your type of cabbage. Kale, for example, only takes about 5 minutes.

Drain and transfer to warm bowls. Add the Parmesan and a twist of black pepper to serve.

SERVES 2

300g (10½oz) hispi, sweetheart or
  pointed cabbage
20g (¾oz) salted butter or olive oil
4 tablespoons water
15g (½oz) Parmesan, finely grated
salt and freshly ground black
  pepper

Per serving 3.7g carbs, 3.3g fibre, 7.6g protein, 17g fat, 208kcal

Curly Kale Pezzi with Tomato Sauce

This is our low-carb version of pasta and tomato sauce. It's just as tasty and quick to prepare with a fraction of the carbs. It's a hit in our restaurants where many customers have switched to pezzi.

Prepare and cook the kale as above.

Meanwhile, heat the tomato sauce in another pan or the microwave until hot. Drain the cabbage and put into warm bowls. Add the sauce and top with the mozzarella, basil leaves, a drizzle of olive oil and a twist of black pepper.

SERVES 2

300g (10½oz) curly kale
20g (¾oz) salted butter or olive oil
4 tablespoons water
½ quantity of Quick Italian Tomato
  Sauce (page 50)
125g (4½oz) mozzarella, roughly
  torn
a few basil leaves
salt and freshly ground black
  pepper

Per serving 11g carbs, 4.7g fibre, 16g protein, 48g fat, 562kcal

White Cabbage Pezzi with Mushroom Cream Sauce

When ribbons of white cabbage are cooked with butter until soft, they make the perfect swap for tagliatelle and are ideal for serving with creamy sauces or ragù.

Cut the cabbage into ribbons and cook it as in the recipe for the Hispi Pezzi (opposite). Toss the drained cabbage with the warmed mushroom cream sauce in the pan and serve in warm bowls.

SERVES 2

300g (10½oz) white cabbage, hard stems removed
20g (¾oz) salted butter or olive oil
4 tablespoons water
1 quantity of Mushroom Cream Sauce (page 58)

Per serving 3.6g carbs, 3.1g fibre, 2.3g protein, 13g fat, 145kcal

Cavolo Nero Pezzi with Bacon, Tomato & Chilli Sauce

The dark, slightly bitter leaves of black kale are softened by the sweet and spicy sauce in this delicious combination. The sauce keeps well for up to five days in the fridge if you want to make a batch of it.

To make the sauce, fry the bacon in the oil for a few minutes in a large frying pan over a medium heat until it starts to brown. Add the garlic, chilli flakes, cherry tomatoes and seasoning and continue to fry for a further 3–4 minutes until the tomatoes soften.

Meanwhile, strip the leaves from the stems of the cavolo nero and tear them into pieces about 5cm (2in) wide. Wash them in cold water and put them into a saucepan with the oil, water and seasoning. Cover and place over a medium heat for about 5 minutes or until the leaves are soft. Taste and adjust the heat and seasoning.

Mix the cabbage with the sauce in the pan or put the sauce on top of the cabbage, scatter over the cheese and serve.

SERVES 2

300g (10½oz) cavolo nero
1 tablespoon extra virgin olive oil
3 tablespoons water

For the bacon, tomato & chilli sauce
4 rashers of streaky bacon, finely chopped
1 tablespoon extra virgin olive oil
1 fat garlic clove, finely chopped
¼–½ teaspoon chilli flakes
10 cherry tomatoes, halved
15g (½oz) Parmesan or Grana Padano, finely grated
salt and freshly ground black pepper

Per serving 6.4g carbs, 4.3g fibre, 26g protein, 34g fat, 445kcal

Broccoli, Ginger & Coconut Soup

This speedy soup can go from chopping board to serving bowl within 15 minutes. We like the crunch of peanuts at the end, but they can be omitted. It is a filling soup that really hits the spot for flavour.

Fry the garlic, ginger, chilli and salt in the coconut oil in a saucepan for a couple of minutes to release their flavour. Add the broccoli stalk and coriander and stir through. After 5 minutes add the florets. Pour in the can of coconut milk, then fill the can with warm water and add this to the pan. Cover and bring to the boil, reduce the heat and let the soup bubble gently for 5–7 minutes or until the broccoli stalks are tender.

Meanwhile, dry-fry the peanuts, if using, until lightly browned, tip onto a board and roughly chop.

Remove the soup from the heat and use a stick blender or food processor to blend it to a smooth consistency. Adjust the seasoning as necessary. Pour into warm bowls and garnish with the coriander leaves, peanuts and black pepper or extra slices of red chilli and with lime wedges alongside for squeezing, if you wish.

SERVES 4

1 garlic clove, roughly chopped
1 heaped tablespoon finely chopped ginger (15g/½oz knob)
¼–½ red chilli, finely chopped, plus extra, thinly sliced, to garnish (optional)
1 teaspoon salt
2 tablespoons coconut oil or ghee
400g (14oz) broccoli, cut into small florets and the stalk thinly sliced
25g (1oz) coriander, stalks and leaves roughly chopped, a few leaves reserved for garnish
1 x 400ml (14fl oz) can of coconut milk
50g (1¾oz) unroasted peanuts (optional)
freshly ground black pepper
lime wedges, to serve (optional)

Per serving 9.2g carbs, 5.5g fibre, 9.2g protein, 31g fat, 361kcal

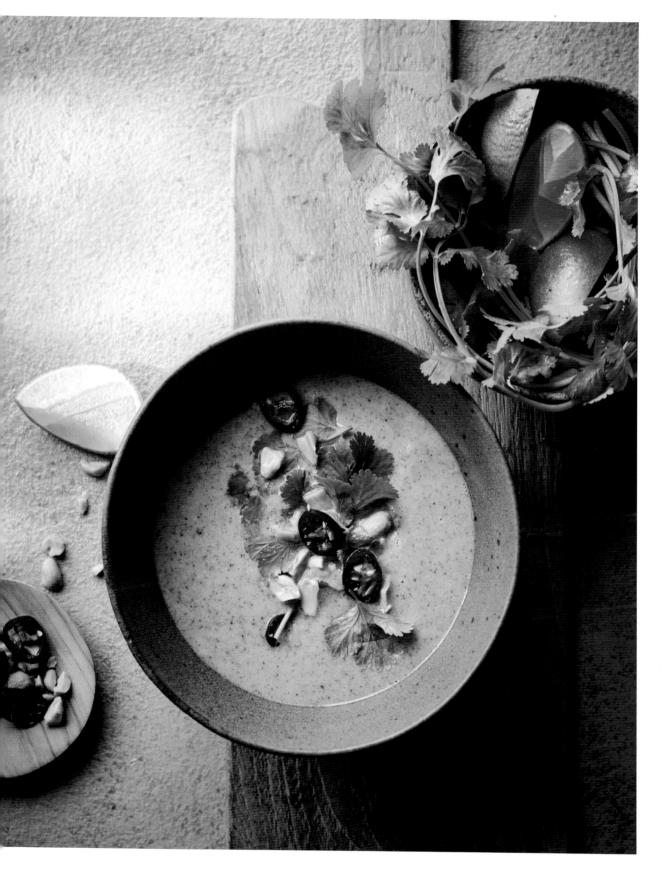

Leek Ribbons with Creamy Chicken & Thyme Sauce

This is a great way to use up leftover chicken from a roast or from making stock. Here we serve it with leek ribbons instead of pasta. It is every bit as delicious but without the bloat and blood sugar highs.

To make the sauce, fry the onion, garlic and seasoning in the butter in a large frying pan over a low heat until soft. Add the chicken and thyme and stir through. Cook for a couple of minutes to heat through, then pour in the wine. Bring to the boil, then reduce the heat to simmer for 5 minutes. Add the cream and stir through. Cook the sauce for a further 5 minutes to thicken. Taste and adjust the seasoning as necessary.

Meanwhile, with your finger, push the centre of the cut leeks to separate the slices into rings. Don't worry if a few stay together. Put the rings into a medium saucepan with a splash of hot water, the butter and seasoning and cover with a lid. Bring to the boil, reduce the heat to simmer for 7–10 minutes until the leeks are tender but still green. Shake the pan frequently during cooking, and if the leeks look dry, add a dash more water.

When the leeks are done, remove the lid and allow any extra water to evaporate. They should be coated in a little buttery glaze. Serve in warm bowls with the creamy chicken on top. Finish with a twist of pepper and a scattering of the Parmesan and parsley.

SERVES 4

*500g (1lb 2oz) leeks, cut into rings
  2cm (¾in) wide
a knob of butter
15g (½oz) Parmesan, finely grated
10g (¼oz) parsley, finely chopped
salt and freshly ground black
  pepper*

For the sauce

*1 onion, finely chopped
1 fat garlic clove, finely chopped
a knob of butter
400g (14oz) cooked chicken,
  roughly chopped
3 sprigs of fresh thyme
100ml (3½fl oz) dry white wine
200ml (7fl oz) double cream*

Per serving 7.2g carbs, 3.3g fibre, 34g protein, 39g fat, 538kcal

Quick Italian Tomato Sauce

In a classic Italian tomato sauce, the onions are slowly sautéed in olive oil first before adding the tomatoes. The sauce is then gently simmered for up to an hour. Great if you have time, if not, in this method it all cooks together, and beats any jar of sauce hands down for its pure, simple ingredients. There are no hidden sugars or preservatives here – just Italian tomatoes, onion and olive oil. Leave it with texture or blend until smooth.

Put all the ingredients in a large frying pan and use a potato masher to break up the tomatoes. Bring the mixture to the boil, then reduce the heat so that the sauce is bubbling rapidly. Cook for about 15 minutes, stirring frequently, until the onions have softened and you are happy with the consistency.

SERVES 6

*5 tablespoons extra virgin olive oil
1 red onion, finely chopped
2 x 400g (14oz) cans of Italian
  plum tomatoes
1 teaspoon salt*

Per serving 5.2g carbs, 1.1g fibre, 1.6g protein, 15g fat, 171kcal

Green Bean "Linguine" with Tuna Puttanesca

Punchy puttanesca brings all the strong flavours of southern Italian cooking to the bowl. In our family we all love it and fight over the last mouthfuls. If you do have leftovers, they can be served cold as a salad the next day. Slice the beans yourself or buy them ready-shredded.

Slice the beans into long lengths using a vegetable peeler, sharp knife or bean slicer. (You can also cut the beans into short lengths, like penne pasta, if you find that easier.) Put the beans into a small saucepan with the butter, a pinch of salt and the water. Cover with a lid and cook over a medium heat for 5–8 minutes or until soft and no longer squeaky against your teeth. Remove the lid and set aside.

Meanwhile, heat the oil in a frying pan, add the tomatoes, olives, garlic, chilli, anchovy fillets and pepper and fry for a couple of minutes until sizzling hot. Add the tuna to the pan and stir through to break it up a little, then add the beans with a couple of tablespoons of any remaining water from the pan. Stir through gently to heat the ingredients and taste for seasoning. Add the parsley, toss through and serve in warm bowls.

SERVES 2

280g (10oz) green, runner or flat beans
a knob of butter
3 tablespoons water
3 tablespoons extra virgin olive oil
10 cherry tomatoes, halved
10 black olives, pitted and halved
1 garlic clove, finely chopped
a pinch of chilli flakes
4 anchovy fillets (optional)
1 x 200g (7oz) can of tuna (150g/5½oz drained weight)
2 tablespoons finely chopped parsley, leaves and stalks
salt and freshly ground black pepper

Per serving 8.6g carbs, 7.1g fibre, 24g protein, 31g fat, 426kcal

Harissa-roasted Cauliflower Steaks with Tahini Dressing & Tomato Salsa

I like to cut the steaks thickly to ensure they stay together and feel substantial enough for a meal. You can only be sure of getting two or three decent steaks from one cauliflower, so do buy the biggest you can find. You can of course use the rest as smaller steaks or make it into Cauli-Rice (see page 66) another day.

Preheat the oven to 240°C/220°C fan/475°F/gas mark 9.

Remove the leaves from the cauliflower and keep for later. Cut away just the tough base of the cauliflower, leaving the central stalk intact. Cut two or three steaks, about 2–3cm (¾–1¼in) thick, from the cauliflower. The florets either side will fall away and can be cooked or saved for Cauli-Rice (see page 66). Lay the steaks on a baking tray with any stray florets if you want to cook them at the same time.

Mix the harissa with the oil and brush it over the steaks, thoroughly coating the surfaces and pushing it into the florets as much as you can. Scatter over a little salt and pepper and then roast for 30–40 minutes or until tender when pierced with a knife and the edges have charred.

Meanwhile, prepare the tahini dressing by mixing the ingredients together in a small bowl. Mix the ingredients for the salsa together in another small bowl. Prepare the cauliflower leaves following the method below and put into the oven just before the end of the cooking time for the steaks.

When the cauliflower is done, remove the tray from the oven and transfer the steaks to serving plates or wooden boards. Arrange as in the photo opposite, or pour the tahini dressing over the steaks, topped with the salsa and the roast cauliflower leaves around the edge.

SERVES 2

1 medium cauliflower, approx. 1kg (2lb 4oz), with leaves and stalk
1 heaped tablespoon harissa paste
3 tablespoons extra virgin olive oil, plus extra for the cauliflower leaves
salt and freshly ground black pepper

For the tahini dressing

2 tablespoons tahini
3 tablespoons water
juice of ½ lemon

For the tomato salsa

2 round tomatoes, finely diced
2 tablespoons roughly chopped coriander
1 tablespoon extra virgin olive oil

Per serving (based on 500g cauliflower) 22g carbs, 7.3g fibre, 11g protein, 38g fat, 485kcal

Roast cauliflower leaves & stems

Preheat the oven to 220°C/200°C fan/425°F/gas mark 7. Rub a little olive oil and seasoning into the leaves and stems and spread them out on a baking tray. Roast for 5–7 minutes or until the leaves become translucent and crisp. Serve warm.

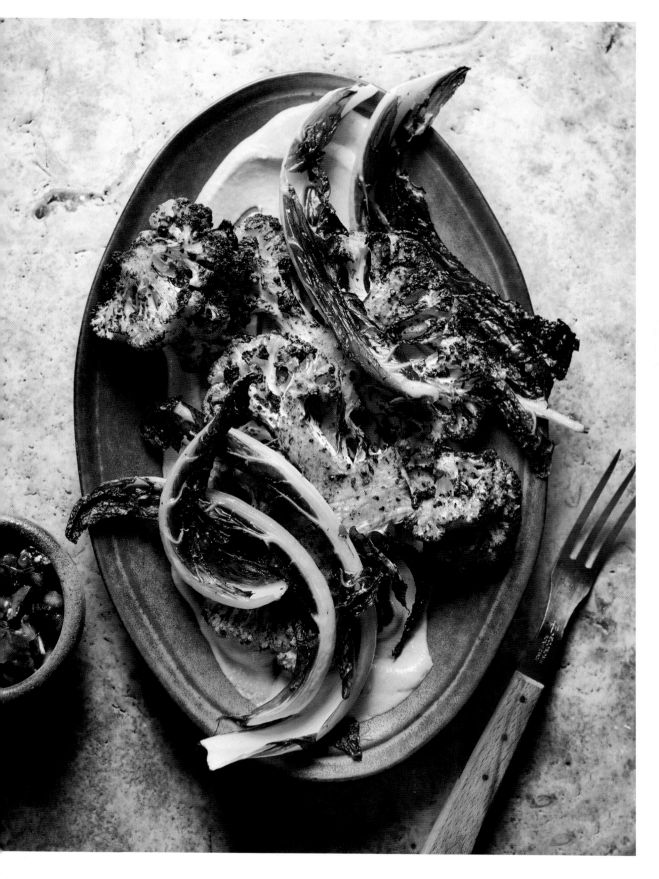

Spiced Red Lentil Soup

This gently spiced soup has all the comfort of a hug from a warm-hearted Indian mamma. Lentils contain both protein and carbohydrate. Our nutritionist Jenny Phillips told me that over one-third of the carbs in lentils is actually indigestible fibre. She explained that the net carbs, which is total carbs minus the fibre, are at an acceptable level for most of us and shouldn't spike blood sugar levels. Our response to carbs is individual, so if you are diabetic you might like to check your blood sugars 30 minutes after eating to see how you respond. When blending the soup, do use a food processor, but cautiously, as you want finely chopped vegetables and not a purée.

Heat the fat in a large saucepan and, when hot, fry the onion, celery, carrot, ginger, garlic, chilli and seasoning together for about 10 minutes over a medium heat or until they have started to soften. Add the spices and cook for a further 2 minutes before adding the lentils and hot water or stock.

Bring the soup to the boil and then reduce the heat so that it bubbles away gently for about 18–20 minutes or until the lentils are soft. Taste and adjust the seasoning with salt, pepper and chilli as necessary. Either roughly purée the soup or leave it as it is with all its lumps, bumps and character.

SERVES 4

3 tablespoons ghee, coconut or extra virgin olive oil
1 medium white onion, finely chopped
1 celery stick, finely chopped
1 medium carrot, finely chopped
2 tablespoons finely chopped ginger
4 garlic cloves, finely chopped
½–1 hot red or green chilli, finely chopped, or ½ teaspoon chilli flakes
1 teaspoon cumin seeds
3 cardamom pods, lightly crushed
1 teaspoon ground turmeric
200g (7oz) dried red lentils
1.5 litres (2¾ pints) hot water or chicken or vegetable stock
salt and freshly ground black pepper

Per serving 31g carbs, 4.2g fibre, 13g protein, 9.8g fat, 272kcal

15-minute Cauliflower Cheese

To cook food "al cartoccio" in Italian means to cook it in a parcel. We love this method, as the flavour of the vegetables is intensified in the enclosed space. It's better than simply steaming because the buttery juices stay in the parcel. The added bonus is that there is less washing up too! Do replace the cauliflower with broccoli, cabbage pezzi (see page 46) or green beans and adjust the cooking times. To add a little crunch, scatter over a few toasted almond slivers as you serve.

Preheat the oven to 200°C/fan 180°C/400°F/gas mark 6.

Cut the cauliflower into even, bite-size florets and the stalk into smaller pieces and slice the leaves and stems.

To make a cartoccio, or parcel, cut a piece of baking parchment at least 10cm (4in) larger than the food you are about to cook. Lay the cauliflower in the centre of the paper, dot with the butter, season and add the water to the parcel to help the steam form. Fold the long ends up to meet each other above the food, then fold again. Do this several times until the fold is about 4cm (1½in) above the food. Now twist the short ends like a sweet wrapper. Place the parcel on a baking tray and cook for 15 minutes.

Meanwhile, make the cheese sauce by heating the cream and Parmesan together in a small saucepan over a medium heat. You can also do this in the microwave in brief bursts. Stir constantly, and as soon as the cheese has melted and the sauce is piping hot, remove it from the heat. It can be easily reheated as you need it.

Remove the cartoccio from the oven and open the parcel, being careful of the hot steam. Serve the cauliflower in the parcel or transfer it to a warm serving dish. Pour over the hot sauce and add a twist of black pepper.

SERVES 2

400g (14oz) cauliflower florets, stalk and leaves
15g (½oz) butter
1 tablespoon water
a pinch of salt and plenty of freshly ground black pepper

For the Parmesan cheese sauce

75ml (2½fl oz) double cream
60g (2¼oz) Parmesan, pecorino or manchego, finely grated

Per serving 15g carbs, 3.6g fibre, 16g protein, 35g fat, 437kcal

Kathryn's Super-simple Stir-fry

This easy but glorious combo comes from our friend Kathryn Tipping and wonderful Peruvian chef Harry Goicochea, who both showed me a similar dish. Kathryn's choice is chicken, broccoli and balsamic while Harry uses lean beef fillet, tomatoes and red wine vinegar to make Lomo Saltado, a traditional Peruvian dish, so vary your veggies according to what you have in the fridge. Both combine soy sauce and vinegar to speedily achieve a rich savouriness to coat the ingredients. This is quick to make once you get cooking, so do have all your ingredients prepped and ready before you start.

Let the oil become hot in a large saucepan or a wok over a high heat. Cook the chicken or beef, stirring, until lightly browned on all sides. Add the ginger and garlic and cook for a minute, stirring constantly.

Add the vegetables and stir well. Cook for 5 minutes or until any water from the vegetables has evaporated and the chicken is cooked through. Add the soy sauce and vinegar, stir and cook for a minute. Taste and season accordingly. Serve scattered with the sesame seeds and coriander, if using.

SERVES 2

2 tablespoons groundnut oil, ghee or coconut oil
2 boneless, skinless chicken breasts or lean beef (weighing approx. 240g/8½oz), cut into even, bite-size pieces
2 garlic cloves, finely chopped
20g (¾oz) ginger, peeled and finely chopped
1 red or yellow pepper, finely sliced
1 onion, finely sliced into half moons
150g (5½oz) broccoli, cut into florets, or cherry tomatoes, halved
1 tablespoon dark soy sauce
1 tablespoon balsamic or red wine vinegar
1 tablespoon sesame seeds, toasted (optional)
a small handful coriander sprigs (optional)
salt and freshly ground black pepper

Per serving 16g carbs, 7.1g fibre, 45g protein, 25g fat, 482kcal

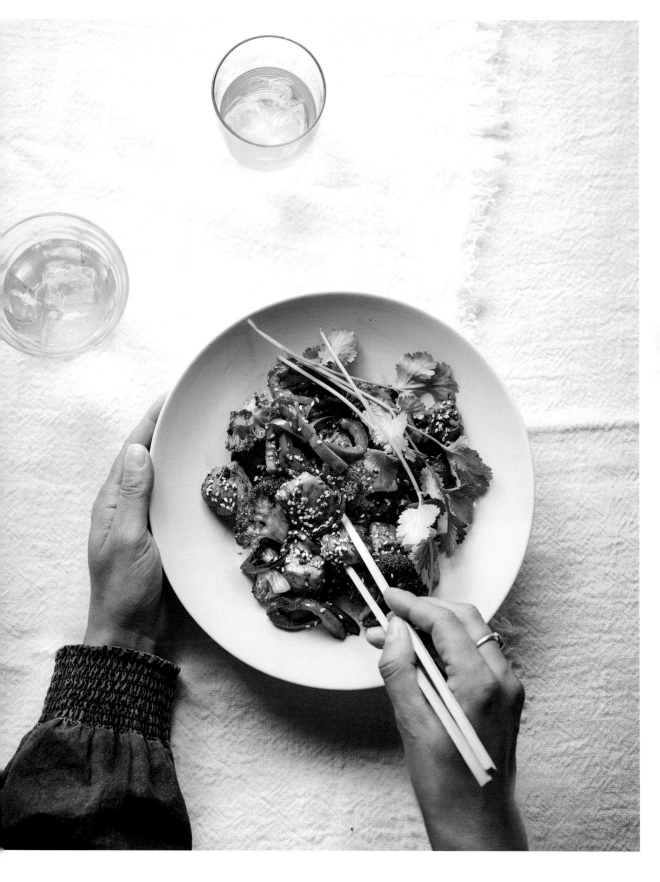

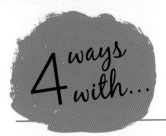

4 ways with... STEAK

On our cookery courses, many people ask why home-cooked steak doesn't taste like one cooked in a restaurant. Apart from the quality of the meat and hanging time, it is often the simple fact that the hand of a chef will be more generous with the salt than that of a home cook. I like to cook sirloin steaks in their own fat for flavour, so do try to buy them with an edge of creamy fat still attached.

Jenny Phillips suggests using saturated animal fat for other cuts, such as lard, dripping or ghee, as they have a lower smoke point than other oils and are not refined or ultra-processed – so do as your grandmother did and collect the fat after roasting meat to re-use. Giancarlo loves ribeye, I like sirloin and both of us love bavette, as it is less expensive and has plenty of flavour.

Steak with Mushroom Cream Sauce

Prepare the sauce first as it can easily be reheated at the last minute to pour over the steak. Heat the oil in a large heavy-based frying pan over a medium heat, add the shallot and garlic and fry for about 7 minutes or until soft but not browned. Add the mushrooms, herbs and seasoning and fry for 10–15 minutes until soft and most of the water from them has evaporated.

Pour in the brandy and sizzle for a couple of minutes until the strong smell of alcohol has dissipated. Discard the herbs. Add the crème fraîche and stir through until hot. Remove from the heat while you cook the steak.

Season the steaks generously with salt and pepper. Warm a non-stick frying pan over a medium-high heat. Hold the two steaks together with tongs with the fat-edge-side down onto a hot frying pan. Let the fat sizzle, brown and melt; you will soon have a pool of it large enough to cook the steaks. Now lay the steaks down separately and cook them to your liking (see page 60).

Serve the steak with the reheated sauce poured over the top.

SERVES 2

2 sirloin steaks with fat along one edge, approx. 450g (1lb) in total
salt and freshly ground black pepper

For the mushroom cream sauce

3 tablespoons extra virgin olive oil
1 shallot or ½ onion, finely chopped
2 garlic cloves, lightly crushed
150g (5½oz) chestnut mushrooms, finely sliced
2 sprigs of thyme and/or a long sprig of rosemary
½ teaspoon salt
a good twist of freshly ground black pepper
3 tablespoons brandy, white wine or sherry vinegar
6 tablespoons crème fraîche or double cream

Per serving (steak) 0g carbs, 0g fibre, 53g protein, 7.6g fat, 280kcal
Per serving (mushroom cream sauce) 5.6g carbs, 1.6g fibre, 4.1g protein, 41g fat, 455kcal

Steak Tagliata with Rocket, Parmesan & Balsamic Dressing

This is an Italian classic where the steaks are cut "tagliata" (sliced) after resting which allows the salt and balsamic vinegar to seep inside the meat. I love to eat it with my fingers from a wooden carving board (with a groove around the outside), taking a few rocket leaves and a crumbly sliver of Parmesan with every slice of steak.

Cook the steaks as in the basic method opposite, using the dripping instead of the rendered fat. Arrange the rocket leaves on a wooden carving board or serving plate. When the steak is cooked to your liking (see page 60), remove it from the pan and let it rest on a wooden board or a warm plate for 5 minutes. Cut it into slices 2cm (¾in) thick using a steak or serrated knife.

Push a slice or a cook's knife under the sliced steak and transfer it to the rocket, keeping each steak as close to its original shape as possible. Drizzle over the olive oil and vinegar, give them both a good twist of pepper and scatter over the Parmesan. Serve straight away.

SERVES 2

2 rib-eye steaks, approx. 450g (1lb) in total
1 tablespoon beef dripping, lard or ghee
40g (1½oz) rocket leaves
2 tablespoons extra virgin olive oil
balsamic vinegar, to drizzle
20g (¾oz) Parmesan, freshly shaved
salt and freshly ground black pepper

Per serving 0.7g carbs, 0.5g fibre, 57g protein, 30g fat, 504kcal

Bavette Steak with Phil's Mexican Rub

This simple but punchy rub comes from Lou and Phil Ford, my sister and her husband, who live in the US. This is one of their favourite steaks to cook. The rub works on any cut of steak, giving a spicy crust to the meat; they serve it with peppers, onions and guacamole.

Mix together the ingredients for the rub in a small bowl. Coat the steak with the rub and lay on a plate. Cover and put into the fridge for up to 30 minutes. Remove the steak and pat off any excess rub. Cook as for the Bavette Steak with Chimichurri (see overleaf).

While the meat is resting, add the vegetables to the meat juices and fat in the pan. Stir-fry the vegetables briefly so that they retain their crunch. Slice the meat thinly against the grain and serve straight away.

SERVES 2

approx. 500g (1lb 2oz) bavette steak, trimmed
1 tablespoon fat, such as goose, duck, beef dripping or lard
1 red or yellow pepper, thinly sliced
1 small onion, sliced

For the rub
1 teaspoon chilli powder
1 teaspoon paprika
1 teaspoon garlic powder
1 teaspoon ground cumin
½ teaspoon dried oregano
1 teaspoon sea salt
¼ teaspoon freshly ground black pepper

Per serving 5.8g carbs, 2.4g fibre, 54g protein, 33g fat, 538kcal

Bavette Steak with Chimichurri

Bavette, also known as flank steak, is from the belly of the calf. It needs to be cooked medium rare for best results and should be cut thinly to serve. It lends itself to barbecuing too, and takes well to a marinade or rub; for both flavour and value it is ideal.

Marinades can't penetrate the meat by any more than a few millimetres, so there is no need to leave it for any longer than 30 minutes–1 hour. Salt in a marinade will allow the other flavours in the marinade to enter the meat, but don't leave it longer than 24 hours or it will begin to cure it. You always need fat and acid too, so as well as oil, lemon juice, vinegar or yogurt will help to tenderize the meat. This vibrant, fresh chimichurri sauce from South America is equally wonderful on steak, chicken, lamb or roast vegetables.

Put the bavette into a dish with the marinade ingredients. Make sure the steak is coated in the marinade, then cover and leave in the fridge for 30 minutes–1 hour maximum. Remove from the dish and allow any marinade to drip off.

Meanwhile, prepare the chimichurri sauce by chopping the herbs, garlic and chilli together on a board. Put into a small bowl and stir through the oil, vinegar and seasoning to taste.

Heat a frying pan to hot over a high heat. Add the fat, and once it has melted and is hot enough to sizzle a piece of bread, put the steak into the pan and fry for 4 minutes a side for medium rare. Remove from the pan and let it rest for 5 minutes before slicing it finely across the grain. Pour over the sauce and serve straight away.

SERVES 4

approx. 1kg (2lb 4oz), bavette steak, trimmed
1 tablespoon fat, such as goose, duck, beef dripping, tallow or lard

For the marinade

4 tablespoons extra virgin olive oil
1 tablespoon salt
1 tablespoon lemon juice

For the chimichurri sauce

10g (¼oz) parsley or coriander, or a mixture of the two, finely chopped
1 small garlic clove, finely chopped
¼–½ red chilli, finely chopped
4 tablespoons extra virgin olive oil
1 tablespoon red or white wine vinegar
salt and freshly ground black pepper

Per serving 0.5g carbs, 0g fibre, 53g protein, 33g fat, 509kcal

How to tell when steak is done

A 2cm- (¾in)-thick sirloin or ribeye steak will take about 1½ minutes a side for rare, 2 minutes a side for medium rare and 3 minutes a side for medium.

To tell when a steak is done to your liking, press the top of it while it is still in the pan. The resistance to touch will demonstrate how it is cooked. You can compare the feeling to various parts of your hand, using this simple guide: Press your thumb and index finger together and prod the soft fleshy area at the base of your thumb with the index finger of your other hand. It will be soft to the touch like a rare steak feels. Next, move your middle finger to touch your thumb and feel the point again – it will feel like a medium rare steak. The third finger will make it feel like 'medium' and the little finger like well done.

Ideally, cooked meat should be rested for the same length of time as it takes to cook. This is because when meat is cooked the juices move to the inside of the meat, causing the outside to become dry. Allowing meat to rest means that they are evenly distributed through the meat again, dispelling any dryness.

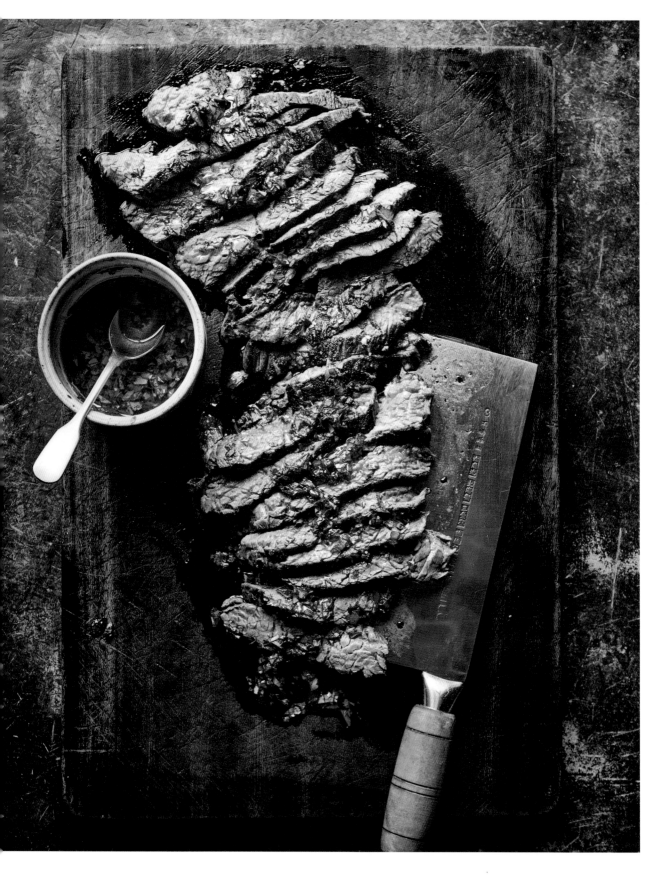

Confit Duck Salad

Warm confit duck must be one of life's luxuries. I expect most of us have walked past cans of it in the aisle of every supermarket and not given it a thought. However, it is traditional to buy it in jars or cans in France and this is why: it makes a deliciously unctuous salad, full of flavour and crispy bits, and gives you the bonus of extra duck fat for cooking afterwards. Once the duck is cooked and shredded, one can goes a long way, so it is not an expensive meal to make. It is also great with any of the vegetable mash recipes on pages 160–161.

Preheat the oven to 240°C/220°C fan/475°F/gas mark 9.

Put the duck pieces, coated in a little fat from the can, onion and garlic cloves on a baking tray and cook for 25–30 minutes. Add the olives to the tray after 15 minutes.

Meanwhile, cook the green beans in boiling salted water for about 7 minutes or until just soft. Drain and set aside.

Make the dressing by mixing the ingredients in a small heatproof bowl.

When the duck is crispy and hot all the way through, transfer it to a chopping board. Pour 100ml (3½fl oz) of the hot cooking juices into the dressing in the bowl and stir through. Pop the garlic out of its skin, mash it to a pulp on the chopping board with a sharp knife or fork and add it to the dressing. Taste the dressing and adjust the seasoning accordingly.

Tear the duck into thick shreds with two forks and toss with the beans, olives and salad leaves. Pour over the dressing and serve straight away.

SERVES 4

425g (15oz) confit duck, drained weight from a 765g (1lb 10½oz) can
1 medium brown or red onion, sliced into half moons
2 fat garlic cloves, unpeeled and lightly crushed
50g (1¾oz) black olives, pitted
200g (7oz) green beans, trimmed
200g (7oz) mixed salad leaves
salt and freshly ground black pepper

For the dressing
2 tablespoons balsamic vinegar
1 tablespoon finely chopped rosemary
1 heaped teaspoon Dijon mustard

Per serving 7.8g carbs, 3.9g fibre, 24g protein, 44g fat, 531kcal

Calves' Liver with Butter & Sage

This classic Italian dish is a brilliant meal in under 3 minutes, which makes this a great choice for a quick supper. The ultimate fast food. And did you know that calves' liver contains more vitamin C, weight for weight, than an apple? Calves' liver is a superfood, as it contains more nutrients (particularly if it's grass-fed) than most other foods and we should be eating more of it. At our restaurants, calves' liver is the biggest-selling dish on our menu; I believe one of the reasons for this is that people don't like to cook it at home. So, the ease of Giancarlo's recipe below might just change that.

Season the liver on both sides. Heat the olive oil in a large non-stick frying pan over a medium heat, add the garlic and fry until it just starts to colour. Increase the heat to high and add the liver pieces to the pan. Fry for 30 seconds on each side for medium-cooked liver (or about 45 seconds on each side for well done). If your pan isn't big enough, fry the liver in two batches. Reduce the heat, add the butter and sage leaves to the pan and continue cooking the liver until the butter has melted.

Serve immediately, dressed with the butter, sage and garlic with celeriac mash (see page 160) or sautéed spinach.

SERVES 4

4 pieces of calves' liver, approx. 150g (5½oz each)
4 tablespoons olive oil
4 garlic cloves, peeled and lightly crushed
75g (2¾oz) salted butter, at room temperature
8 large sage leaves
salt and freshly ground black pepper

Per serving 0.6g carbs, 0g fibre, 28g protein, 35g fat, 410kcal

Pork Shogayaki with Shredded Cabbage

Ultra-thin slices of pork in a ginger and soy sauce is a simple Japanese dish frequently cooked at home or found in bento boxes prepared and sold at railways stations for hungry passengers. Shogayaki is nearly always sold with finely shredded cabbage, which is surprisingly tasty for such a simple addition, as it helps to mop up the sauce on the plate. Although not Japanese, I like to toss the cabbage in a tiny drizzle of toasted sesame oil but Giancarlo likes his plain; the choice is yours. You can use any lean cut of pork, chicken or turkey for this dish, but do make sure there is no sinew and, when bashing the meat, do keep the slices very thin and even.

Make up the sauce by mixing the ingredients together in a small bowl.

Put the pork under a piece of plastic film (that from a bunch of flowers is ideal – don't use clingfilm) and bash out with a meat tenderizer to a thickness of 3mm (⅛in). Heat the oil in a large non-stick frying pan and, when hot enough to sizzle a tiny piece of the meat, fry the pork escalopes for 1–2 minutes a side or until cooked through.

Remove the pork from the pan and put onto a warm plate. Pour away the excess oil and put the pork back. Now pour the sauce over the meat and into the pan. Let it bubble for a minute and then turn the meat on the other side for a further minute. When the sauce has reduced slightly and is piping hot, it is ready to serve on plates with the cabbage alongside. Scatter over the sesame and nigella, if using, seeds and serve straight away.

SERVES 4

300g (10½oz) pork escalopes
1 tablespoon groundnut or olive oil
150g (5½oz) white cabbage, very finely shredded
1 tablespoon toasted black and/or white sesame seeds
1 teaspoon nigella seeds (optional)

For the sauce

6 tablespoons sake or rice wine
3 tablespoons mirin
3 tablespoons soy sauce
30g (1oz) ginger, peeled and grated
2 garlic cloves, grated

Per serving 22g carbs, 3.1g fibre, 36g protein, 15g fat, 431kcal

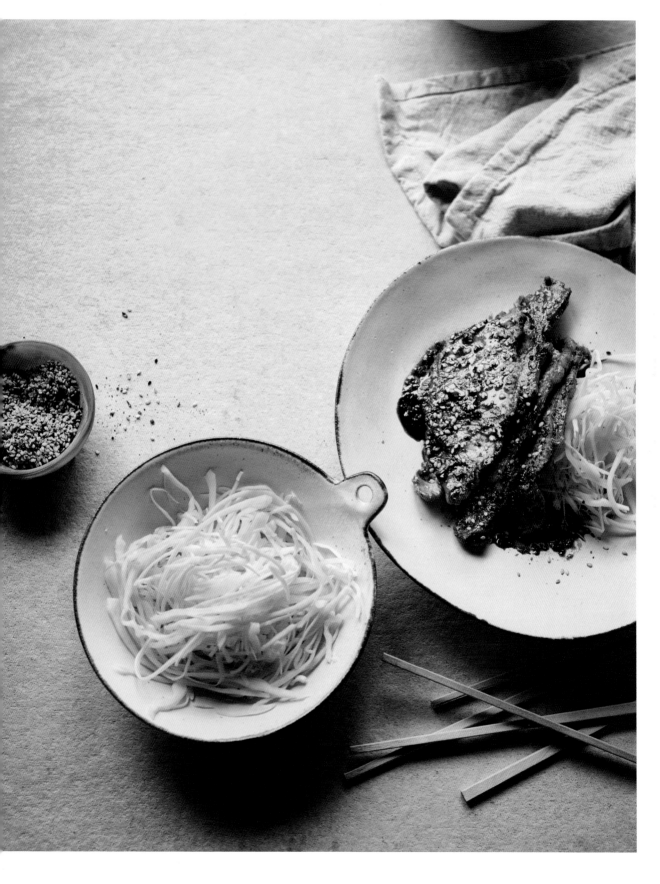

4 ways with... CAULI-RICE

To avoid the spikes of glucose in your bloodstream from eating any kind of rice, switch to cauli-rice. It takes just minutes to prepare and has endless flavour possibilities that can be added if you stir-fry it. It keeps well in the fridge for up to 3 days (or in the freezer for up to 3 months), so leftovers are quick to reheat. You can also use broccoli or sprouts in the same way. Once riced, the vegetables expand in volume – you need to allow about 150g (5½oz) cauli-rice per person.

For Basic Cauli-Rice

This simple recipe will match any food; leave it as it is or embellish it as you like with herbs or spices.

Cut the head of the cauliflower into large florets and roughly chop the stalk and leaves. Put one-third of the cauliflower into a food processor and pulse until finely chopped (it will resemble large grains of rice), making sure you don't end up with a purée. Tip the cauliflower into a bowl and repeat with the remaining two-thirds. If you don't have a food processor, coarsely grate the florets and stalk and finely chop the leaves.

Heat the oil in a wok or large frying pan. Fry the onion over a medium heat for 7 minutes or until soft. Add the cauliflower rice, season and stir through. Add the water, cover and cook over a low heat for 5–7 minutes or until just soft, stirring occasionally.

SERVES 4

600g (1lb 5oz) cauliflower florets, stalk and leaves
3 tablespoons extra virgin olive oil, ghee, coconut oil, chicken fat or beef dripping
1 onion or 5 spring onions, finely chopped
1 teaspoon salt
3 tablespoons water
freshly ground black pepper

Per serving 13g carbs, 3.5g fibre, 10g fat, 4.1g protein, 162kcal

Turmeric Cauli-Rice

We love this with Middle Eastern food and curries. For presentation points and a little crunch, add a few toasted slivered almonds.

Follow the basic recipe for Cauli-Rice above, adding the garlic, spices and chilli at the same time you fry the onion. Taste and adjust the seasoning. Stir in the coriander, if using, just before serving.

SERVES 4

1 quantity of Basic Cauli-Rice (above)
2 garlic cloves, lightly crushed
1 small cinnamon stick
4 cardamom pods, split
½ teaspoon ground turmeric
a pinch of chilli flakes, to taste
a few sprigs of coriander, leaves picked and stalks finely chopped (optional)
salt and plenty of freshly ground black pepper

Per serving 14g carbs, 3.6g fibre, 4.2g protein, 10g fat, 163kcal

Orange & Harissa Cauliflower Couscous

This amber-coloured and orange-scented rice is perfect with the Lamb Shank Tagine on page 140 or with simply grilled lamb chops or roasted chicken pieces. Keep it simple with the spice and harissa or bejewel it with pomegranate seeds as we did on the photo on page 141.

Roast the pine nuts in a dry frying pan over a medium heat until lightly browned. Tip out of the pan and leave to cool.

Follow the basic recipe for Cauli-Rice opposite, adding the garlic, chilli and spices to the onions after they have softened. Let them cook for a couple of minutes. Add the cauli-rice, seasoning, harissa, 1 teaspoon of orange zest and water. Cover and cook for 5–7 minutes or until soft, stirring occasionally. Taste and adjust the seasoning and orange zest as necessary.

Stir in the herbs and pine nuts, scatter over the pomegranate seeds, if using, and serve straight away.

SERVES 4

3 tablespoons pine nuts
1 quantity of Basic Cauli-Rice (opposite)
3 garlic cloves, finely chopped
¼–½ teaspoon chilli flakes
1 teaspoon ground cumin
½ teaspoon ground turmeric
2 tablespoons harissa paste
1–2 teaspoons finely grated orange zest
4 tablespoons water
a large handful of coriander and/or parsley, leaves roughly chopped, stalks finely chopped
100g (3½oz) pomegranate seeds (optional)
salt and freshly ground black pepper

Per serving 18g carbs, 5g fibre, 6.2g protein, 17g fat, 250kcal

Sausage Ragù & Cauli-Rice Pilaf

Pilaf, a Middle Eastern dish mainly associated with Turkey and a cousin of Indian pilau, is normally made with rice, but this version halves the carbs and packs in the flavour. It is a great way to use up leftover roast meat, such as the Mechoui Leg of Lamb on page 144, vegetables like the Italian Roast Vegetables on page 68 or sauces, such as ragù or the mushroom cream sauce on page 58, or any of the tomato sauces in the book (see page 50).

Heat the sausage ragù in a large frying pan.

Prepare the cauli-rice as in the basic recipe opposite. Add to the ragù, stir the two together and serve straight away.

SERVES 4

1 quantity of Sausage Ragù (page 146)
1 quantity of Basic Cauli-Rice (opposite)

Per serving 20g carbs, 5.3g fibre, 34g protein, 42g fat, 619kcal

Oven-baked Fish in Paper Parcel with Capers, Olives & Tomatoes

Serve the fish with a glass of white wine, some green beans dressed with your best olive oil and you will feel like you are in Italy by the sea.

Preheat the oven to 200°C/180°C fan/400°F/gas mark 6.

Lay the fish on a piece of baking parchment about 10cm (4in) larger than the fish on all sides. Season and then scatter over the tomatoes, olives, capers and oregano. Pour over the oil and white wine.

Bring the long edges of the paper together to meet each other above the fish, then fold them over by 2cm (¾in). Do this again and again until you they reach about 5cm (2in) above the fish. Twist the ends like a sweet wrapper to seal in the steam and flavours. Lay the parcel on a baking tray and bake for 12–15 minutes or until the fish is cooked through. It should feel firm through the paper when it is done. Serve warm in the paper on a serving plate scattered with the parsley.

SERVES 2

450g (1lb) haddock, cod, whiting or other firm white fish fillet
6 cherry tomatoes, halved
8 black or green olives, pitted
2 tablespoons small capers, drained
½ teaspoon dried oregano
2 tablespoons extra virgin olive oil
2 tablespoons white wine
a few sprigs of parsley, roughly chopped
salt and freshly ground black pepper

Per serving 1.7g carbs, 0.7g fibre, 41g protein, 14g fat, 311kcal

Italian Roast Vegetables

Here is our staple recipe for roasting vegetables Italian style. Always tuck the herbs under the vegetables to give flavour and stop them burning on the base of the tin, and space the vegetables out so that they all roast rather than steam in a pile.

Preheat the oven to 220°C/200°C fan/425°F/gas mark 7. Grease a baking tray (or two) with a little of the olive oil and lay the rosemary sprigs in it.

Put the vegetables into a bowl with the remaining olive oil, garlic and seasoning and toss to combine. Spread them evenly over the tray(s) in one layer. Cook for 30 minutes until cooked through and golden brown on top.

SERVES 6

4 tablespoons extra virgin olive oil
2 sprigs of rosemary, left whole
1 aubergine, cut lengthways into slices 1cm (½in) thick
1 courgette, sliced into rings 1cm (½in) thick
1 red or yellow pepper, cut into 2cm (¾in) strips
1 onion, cut into 2cm (¾in) wedges
2 garlic cloves, unpeeled and lightly crushed
a large pinch of salt and freshly ground black pepper

Per serving 7.1g carbs, 4g fibre, 2.2g protein, 13g fat, 162kcal

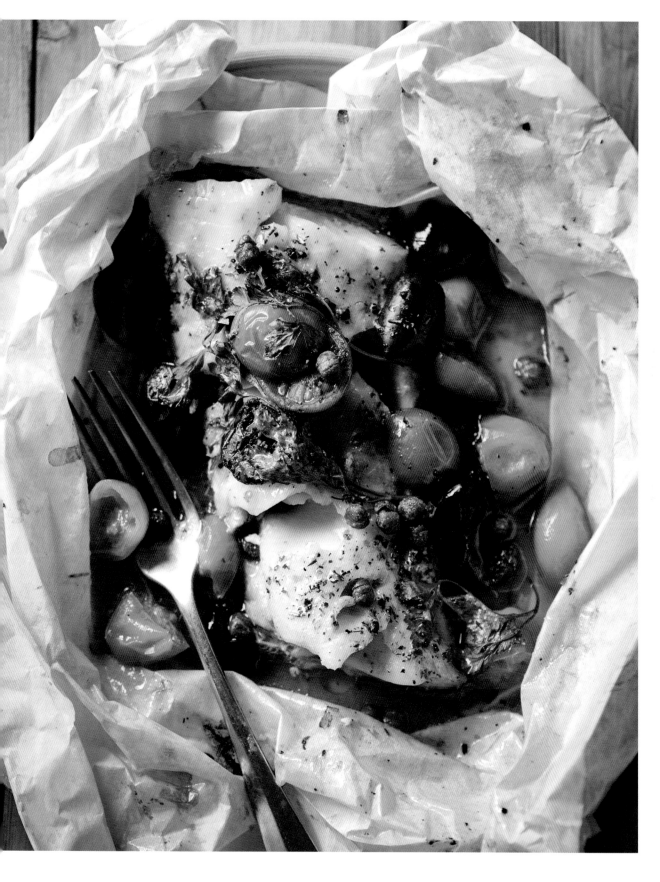

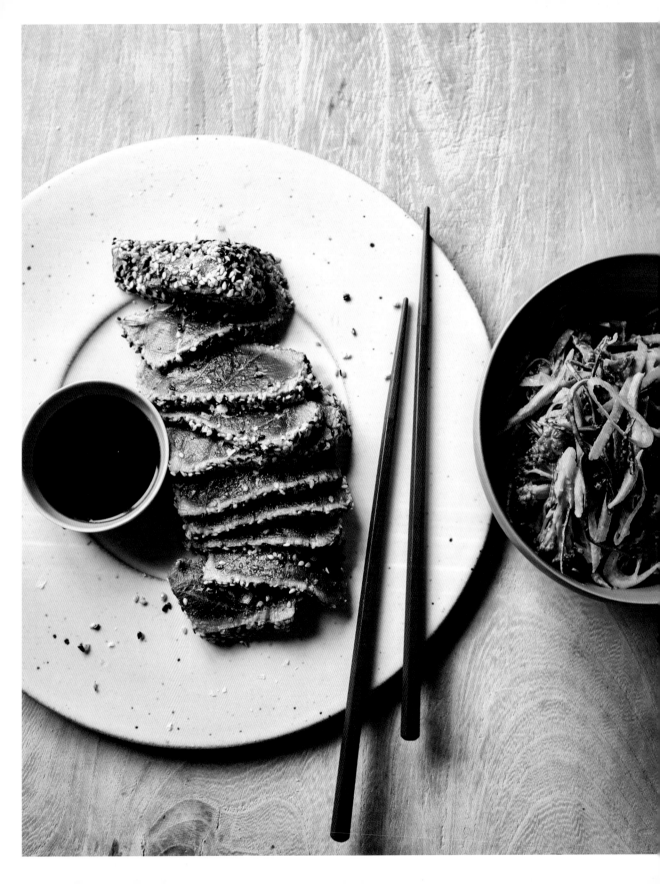

Sesame-crusted Tuna with Ponzu Sauce & Seaweed, Carrot & Broccoli Salad

Commercially frozen or sushi-grade are the safest options for eating tuna rare. This recipe is inspired by Japanese cookery specialist Shirley Booth. She suggests using lemon and lime juice instead of yuzu juice for the ponzu as it is hard to find a good yuzu juice outside Japan. Any leftover ponzu is good for salads or thinly sliced steak.

Seaweed differs from bland-but-pretty arame to the seawater-tasting wakame, so assorted packs are best for a range of texture, colour and nutrition. The salad dressing is traditionally made in a suribachi, a ridged pestle and mortar, but a standard one does the trick or use tahini instead. Leftover sauce is perfect with green beans and boiled eggs.

Toasted sesame oil, my addition, is not good for frying, so I brush it onto the tuna before serving. Speed up cutting the vegetables by using a food processor.

For the salad, rehydrate the seaweed according to the packet instructions; normally this is between 10–30 minutes. Put the vegetables into a bowl and cover with just-boiled salted water. Leave to stand for 4 minutes, then drain and plunge them into a bowl of ice-cold water.

To make the sauce for the salad, toast the seeds, if using, in a dry frying pan until golden. Transfer to a sheet of paper to cool. Shoot the seeds from the paper into a pestle and mortar and grind to a powdery paste. Mix this, or the tahini, with the mirin and soy sauce, and add the cold water to dilute into a creamy pouring sauce. Taste and add salt if necessary.

Drain the seaweed and vegetables, then toss with the sauce in a bowl ready to serve or keep at room temperature for a couple of hours if you need to prepare it first.

Make the ponzu sauce by mixing the ingredients together in a bowl.

Pat the tuna steaks dry with kitchen paper and season them all over with salt. Put the sesame seeds on a plate and dip the tuna steaks into the seeds to coat them on all sides.

Heat the groundnut oil in a frying pan over a high heat; it should reach the point where a sesame seed sizzles instantly when dropped into the pan. If you like your tuna very rare, sear the steaks for 30–60 seconds on each side or until the seeds are browned, or for 2 minutes so they are cooked on the outside and rare in the middle. Use tongs to hold the steaks upright to sear the edges briefly. Transfer to a warm serving plate and brush with the toasted sesame oil. Slice and serve with the ponzu sauce and salad.

SERVES 2

2 sustainably caught yellowfin tuna steaks, approx. 200g (7oz) each and about 3cm (1¼in) thick
4 tablespoons black and/or white sesame seeds
2 tablespoons groundnut oil
2 teaspoons toasted sesame oil
salt

For the seaweed, carrot & broccoli salad

10g (¼oz) dried seaweed such as wakame, agar, aka tsunomata and arame
2 spring onions, finely sliced
100g (3½oz) carrots, julienned
100g (3½oz) broccoli, cauliflower or sprouts, finely sliced
50g (1¾oz) Savoy or other green cabbage, finely sliced
4 tablespoons sesame seeds or 3 tablespoons tahini
2 teaspoons mirin
1 tablespoon soy sauce
3–4 tablespoons cold water

For the ponzu sauce

3 tablespoons soy or tamari sauce
1 tablespoon rice or white wine vinegar
1 tablespoon mirin or rice wine
2 tablespoons yuzu juice, or 1 tablespoon lemon juice and 1 tablespoon lime juice

Per serving (tuna) 5.1g carbs, 2.1g fibre, 55g protein, 31g fat, 533kcal
Per serving (salad) 11g carbs, 8.4g fibre, 8.1g protein, 13g fat, 215kcal

Grilled Prawn & Chorizo Traybake

Roll up your sleeves, put finger bowls and some napkins on the table and get stuck into this gloriously colourful platter of garlicky prawns and chorizo. Serve it with the low-carb Rosemary & Olive Rolls (page 101) to mop up the juices. If you are barbecuing, the ingredients can be threaded onto skewers and cooked on the grill.

Preheat the grill to hot. Remove the shell from around the body of the prawns, leaving the head and tail intact.

Put the prawns, chorizo, tomatoes and green pepper in a roasting tray and drizzle over the wine and oil. Season all over and toss everything together with your hands.

Put the tray under the grill for 4–5 minutes or until the prawns become pink. Remove from the grill and turn the prawns over with tongs. Put back under the grill for a further 4–5 minutes or until the prawns are cooked through. Sprinkle with the parsley and serve straight away from the roasting tray (or transfer to a warm platter or a wooden board with a groove around the outside to catch the juices) with the lemon wedges alongside.

SERVES 4

350g (12oz) raw tiger prawns
125g (4½oz) smoked hot chorizo, cut into 1cm (½in) slices
12 cherry tomatoes
1 green pepper, cut into 2cm (¾in) cubes
4 tablespoons dry white wine or dry sherry
4 tablespoons extra virgin olive oil
a small handful of parsley, roughly chopped
salt and freshly ground black pepper
lemon wedges, to serve

Per serving 5.4g carbs, 2.1g fibre, 24g protein, 24g fat, 347kcal

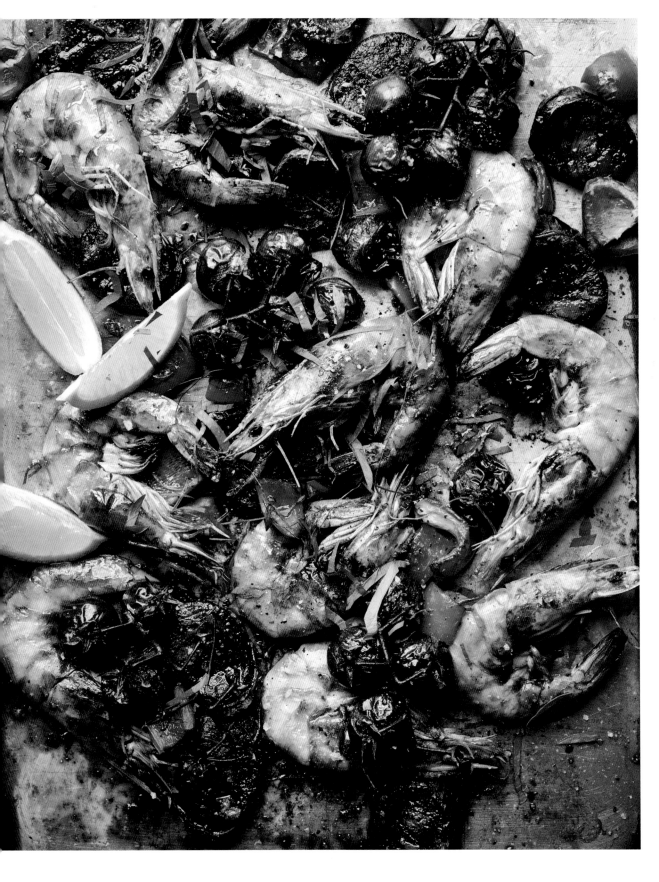

Smoked Mackerel Fishcakes with Horseradish & Lemon Crème Fraîche

Smoked mackerel gives a familiar, traditional taste to the fishcakes and brings all the goodness of oily fish; to vary them, use hot-smoked salmon, canned salmon or sardines. These fishcakes are ideal as a light lunch or supper with crème fraîche and the Green Salad on page 78 with Lemon & Honey Dressing (page 79). To make them more substantial try one as a burger in a Sesame Bun (page 124) with lettuce, tomato and the Horseradish & Lemon Crème Fraîche here, and/or the Robbie's Hot Salsa Roja on page 122. These are also delicious made half the size to serve as canapés.

Preheat the oven to 220°C/200°C fan/425°F/gas mark 7. Grease a baking tray with the oil.

To make the fishcakes, either chop the fish, onions and parsley by hand, mash the lentils with a fork in a bowl and then combine with the remaining ingredients, or put all the ingredients into a food processor and blitz until you have a rough textured paste.

Divide the mixture into 8 balls (each one will weigh roughly 70g/2½oz) and shape into patties about 7cm (2¾in) diameter and 2cm (¾in) thick. Lay them onto the prepared baking tray and cook for 20 minutes or until hot inside and firm to the touch. They should be lightly browned.

Meanwhile, make the horseradish and lemon crème fraîche. Mix the ingredients together briefly in a small bowl, adjust the seasoning to taste and put in the fridge to chill.

Serve the fishcakes warm or at room temperature with the lemon wedges and the horseradish and lemon crème fraîche and the Green Salad (page 78), if you wish.

SERVES 4/MAKES 8 FISHCAKES

1 tablespoon extra virgin olive oil or ghee, to grease
200g (7oz) smoked mackerel fillets, skinned
4 spring onions
3 tablespoons finely chopped parsley
265g (9½oz) cooked or canned, drained Puy or green lentils, cooked from 130g (4½oz) dried lentils
finely grated zest of 1 lemon
1 egg
½ teaspoon salt and plenty of freshly ground black pepper (unless using peppered mackerel)
lemon wedges, to serve

For the horseradish & lemon crème fraîche
juice of ½ lemon
100g (3½oz) crème fraîche
2 tablespoons horseradish sauce
salt and freshly ground black pepper

Per serving 13g carbs, 3.5g fibre, 19g protein, 28g fat, 391kcal

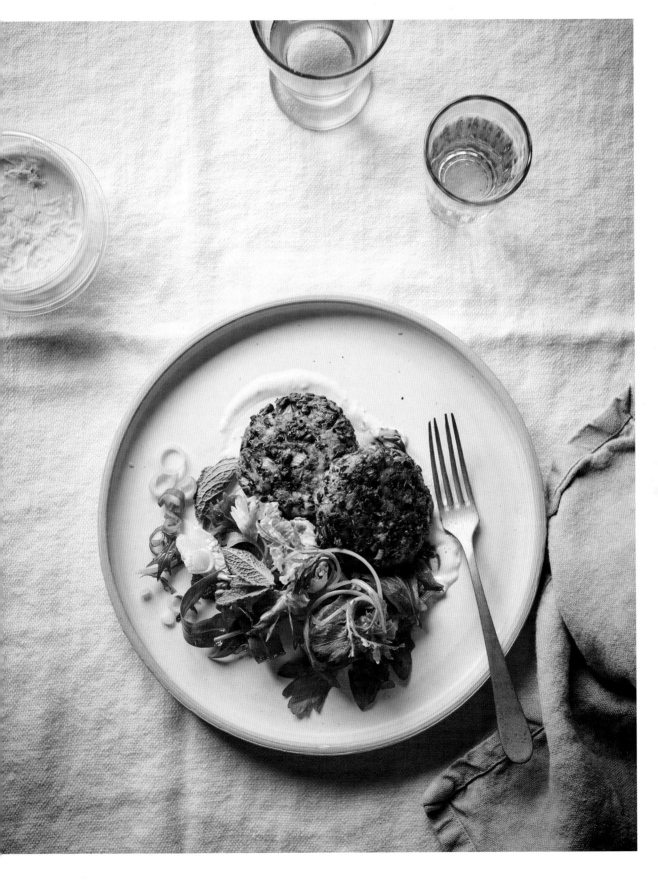

Mexican Sea Bass with Pico de Gallo Salsa

This spicy salsa is one of my favourites and can be used in so many ways. If chopped small it can be a topping for nachos (see page 138) or kept chunky for grilled fish and meats, piled into tacos or packed into small containers for a lunchbox.

Preheat the oven to 240°C/220°C fan/475°F/gas mark 9.

For the salsa, quarter the cherry tomatoes, put them in a sieve over a bowl and sprinkle with ½ teaspoon of salt. Leave to drain for 10 minutes.

Meanwhile, put the spring onions in a bowl of cold water to remove some of their strength.

Season the fish on both sides and lay the fillets in a greased ovenproof dish. Pour over the olive oil and put the fillets into the oven to cook for 8–12 minutes or until firm to the touch and cooked through.

Drain the onions and tip into a mixing bowl with the sieved tomatoes and remaining salsa ingredients. Taste and adjust the seasoning as necessary.

Serve the fish and the salsa, garnished with a few coriander sprigs and a wedge of lime, if you wish.

SERVES 2
4 sea bass fillets or similar fish
2 tablespoons extra virgin olive oil
a few sprigs of coriander, to garnish
lime wedges (optional)

For the pico de gallo salsa
6 cherry tomatoes
3 spring onions or 1 small shallot, finely chopped
2 avocados, cut into bite-size cubes
finely grated zest and juice of 1 lime
½ red, orange, yellow or green pepper, cut into 3cm (1¼in) dice
2 tablespoons extra virgin olive oil
1 small garlic clove, finely chopped
¼–½ green or red chilli, finely chopped
a small handful of coriander leaves, stalks finely chopped
salt and freshly ground black pepper

Per serving 6.8g carbs, 6.8g fibre, 52g protein, 58g fat, 775kcal

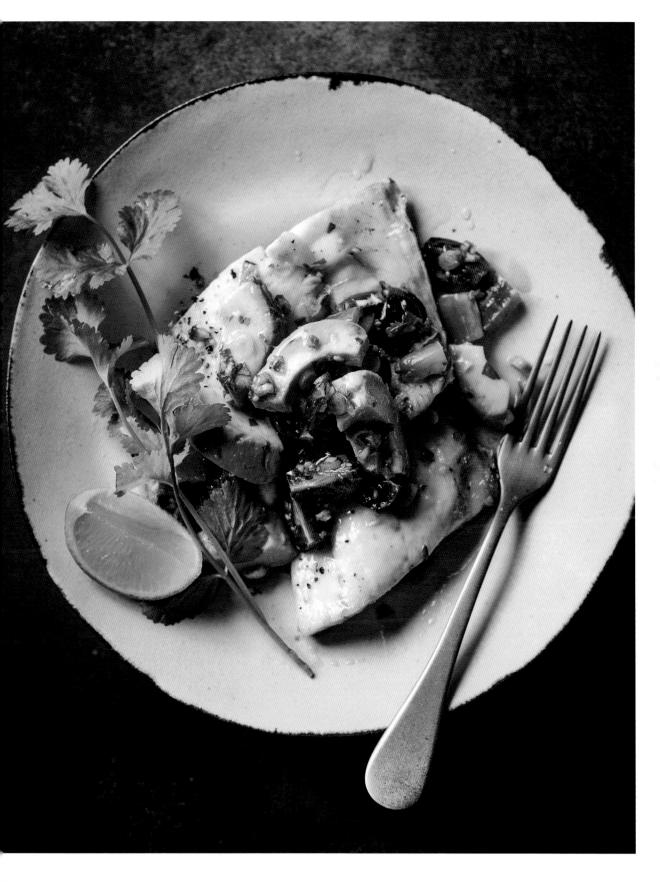

The Green Salad

Salad should never be boring; I'm convinced more people would enjoy salad if it is made with tasty fresh leaves and has a good dressing. For more ideas, have a look at our book *Around the World in Salads*. I like to prepare the cucumber slices into these delicate flower shapes, but do leave the skin on and simply slice if you prefer.

Put the onions into cold water in a small bowl to take away their strength. Toast the seeds in a dry pan until they pop, then tip onto a plate to cool.

Peel the cucumber with a vegetable peeler. Use the prongs of a fork to score down the length of the cucumber, leaving shallow grooves all around it. Now thinly slice it and lay half of the slices over a large serving plate. Add half the lettuce leaves and celery. Roughly tear the celery leaves, mint and parsley and add half of those too. Finely chop the parsley stalks and add. Repeat with the remaining ingredients. The salad will keep like this in the fridge or a cool place for a few hours.

SERVES 4

3 spring onions, finely chopped
1 tablespoon pumpkin seeds
½ English cucumber
250g (9oz) Romaine, Iceberg,
  Baby Gem or soft round lettuce
  leaves, torn into shreds
2 celery sticks, very thinly sliced,
  plus a handful of celery leaves,
  roughly torn
5g (⅛oz) fresh mint leaves
15g (½oz) parsley

Per serving 3.5g carbs, 1.8g fibre, 2.5g protein, 2.3g fat, 47kcal

One-minute Mayonnaise

Take your pick as to which oil to use from the list below, but don't be tempted to use extra virgin olive oil in this mayo, as it is too strong and bitter. Like most homemade mayonnaises, this includes raw egg, so it isn't suitable for pregnant women or anyone in poor health. This is the basic recipe, but you can flavour it with a little grated fresh or mashed roasted garlic, lemon zest, chopped chives, chipotle or curry powder.

Put all the ingredients into the narrow, tall mixing bowl of a stick blender or, if you don't have one, use a narrow, tall jam jar instead. There should only be up to 1cm (½in) of room around the blender stick.

Put the stick blender to the bottom and whizz for 30 seconds or until you see a thick mayonnaise forming. At that point, slowly lift the blender upwards to mix in all of the oil; don't worry if there is a little on top, as you can stir this in.

Now taste the mayo, and at this stage you can stir in more lemon juice, mustard, seasoning or other flavourings. This will keep for up to 3 days in the fridge.

SERVES 4

1 egg
1 heaped teaspoon Dijon mustard
1 teaspoon lemon juice
½ teaspoon salt
a good few twists of black pepper
150ml (¼ pint) avocado,
  macadamia or light olive oil

Per serving 0g carbs, 0.5g fibre, 1.9g protein, 36g fat, 333kcal

Variation
GARLIC MAYONNAISE
This is ideal with the Chicken Shawarma on page 132. Simply add ½–1 teaspoon of grated garlic to the One-minute Mayonnaise to taste.

Jar Dressings

To make the following dressings, put all the ingredients in a jar and shake until emulsified. Keep any remaining dressing in the jar in the fridge for up to a week.

Balsamic & Lemon Dressing

SERVES 4

4 tablespoons extra virgin olive oil
1 tablespoon balsamic vinegar
juice of ½ lemon
½ teaspoon finely grated lemon zest
½ teaspoon Dijon mustard
½ teaspoon salt and plenty of freshly ground black pepper

Per serving 0.6g carbs, 0g fibre, 0g protein, 13g fat, 118kcal

Lemon & Honey Dressing

SERVES 4

4 tablespoons extra virgin olive oil
juice of ½ lemon
½ teaspoon honey
salt and freshly ground black pepper

Per serving 0.7g carbs, 0g fibre, 0g protein, 13g fat, 116kcal

Vinaigrette

SERVES 8

8 tablespoons extra virgin olive oil
2 tablespoons red wine vinegar
1 heaped teaspoon Dijon mustard
1 tablespoon lemon juice
1 small garlic clove, grated
½ teaspoon honey (optional)
½ teaspoon salt
a good pinch of freshly ground black pepper

Per serving 0.5g carbs, 0g fibre, 0g protein, 13g fat, 118kcal

Creamy Vinaigrette

I saw this recipe while looking through historical cookbooks for ideas. It seemed to be the forerunner of mayonnaise and was used over sliced cold meats, vegetables and salad.

To make a creamy vinaigrette, add 4 tablespoons of double cream to the vinaigrette recipe (opposite). Keep stirring until well blended.

Per serving 0.5g carbs, 0g fibre, 0g protein, 17.3g fat, 158kcal

Katie's Top Salad Tips

1 Salad leaves can be splendid used as a single type or mix in celery leaves, watercress, rocket, beetroot leaves, wild mustard, cress or mizuna.

2 Throw in huge handfuls of herbs; they are leaves too.

3 Add texture with seeds, apple, nuts or chopped herb stalks.

4 Serve the dressing on the side – that way, if you have leftover salad it will keep until the next day.

5 Layer it up; it is such a shame when you are the last to arrive at a buffet and the interesting toppings have gone.

6 Serve with tongs; it's easier.

7 Taste your dressing and adjust the balance of sour, salt and heat.

8 Salad shouldn't always reside in a bowl; platters, boards and meat cutting boards with a rim are ideal.

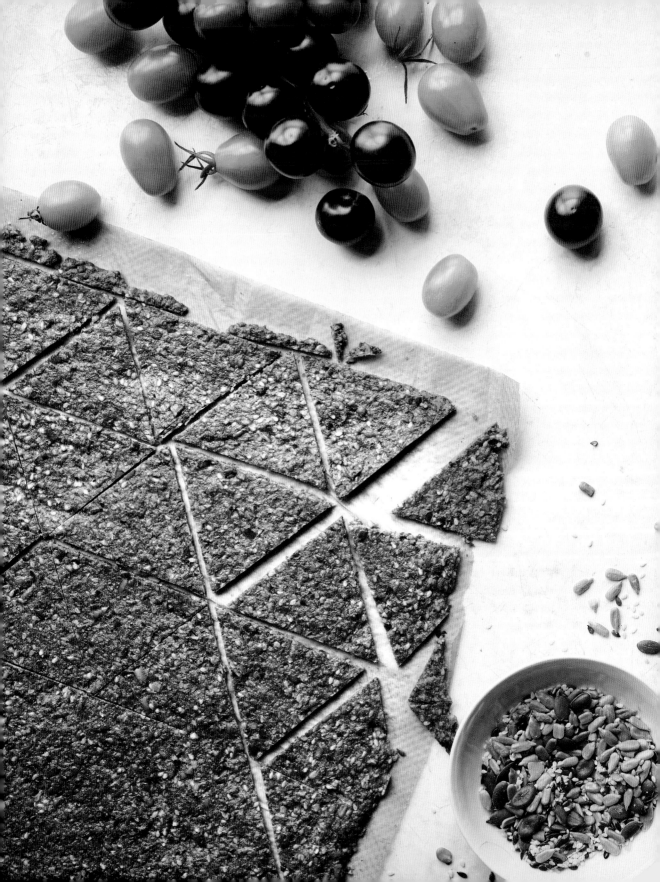

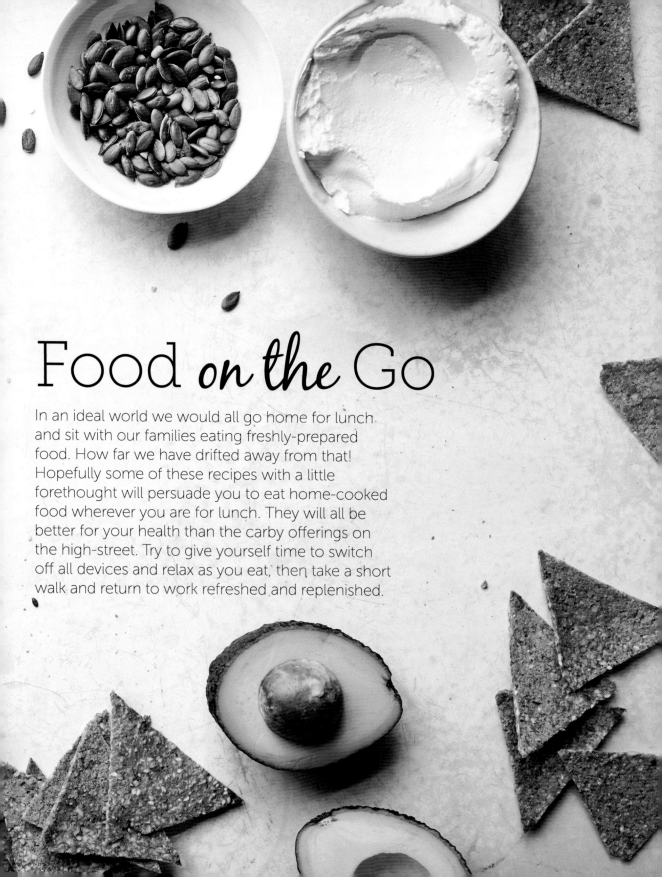

Food *on the* Go

In an ideal world we would all go home for lunch and sit with our families eating freshly-prepared food. How far we have drifted away from that! Hopefully some of these recipes with a little forethought will persuade you to eat home-cooked food wherever you are for lunch. They will all be better for your health than the carby offerings on the high-street. Try to give yourself time to switch off all devices and relax as you eat, then take a short walk and return to work refreshed and replenished.

Mushroom & Noodle Soup

This light, vegan soup has an earthy flavour from the shiitake mushrooms, a hint of sea salt from the kombu (dried kelp) as well as the savoury qualities of miso; it is a soup that nourishes and warms the soul and belly alike. It keeps well in the fridge or in a container for work. I have added konjac noodles to it to give it body. These noodles, also known as shirataki, are made from the konjac root and contain 1.8g carbs per 100g, compared to rice noodles which contain 82g per 100g.

Since my recent travels to Japan to learn Japanese cookery, I have fallen for the earthy, salty-but-sweet charms of miso – fermented soya bean paste – that has a deep savoury flavour. It can be used as a marinade or made into soups or sauces. White miso has a sweet, mild flavour, red miso is punchier and dark miso is robust, as it is fermented for longer. The red is my favourite; it's versatile, with a good strength that gives a savoury umami flavour to everything it touches. A jar will keep in the fridge for up to a year.

Soak the shiitake and kombu in 500ml (18fl oz) of the hot water for at least 3 hours or overnight. As the water cools, they will soften and release their flavour to form a rich, umami stock.

Pour the stock through a sieve into a medium saucepan and add the remaining 1 litre (1¾ pints) of hot water. Pick out the kombu and add it to the pan. Chop the shiitake mushrooms into bite-size pieces and add to the stock. Put all the remaining ingredients, except the noodles and spinach, into the pan and bring to the boil. Reduce the heat to a gentle simmer and cook for 30 minutes. Adjust the seasoning with tamari, miso and chilli to your taste.

Prepare the noodles according to the manufacturer's instructions, then drain, add to the pan with the baby spinach leaves and stir through. Remove the kombu (it can be added to other stock). Serve hot with a spoon for the soup and chopsticks for the noodles.

SERVES 4

20g (¾oz) dried shiitake mushrooms
1 piece of kombu about 5 x 10cm (2 x 4in)
1.5 litres (2¾ pints) hot water
2–3 tablespoons red miso paste
25g (1oz) ginger, peeled and finely sliced
2 celery sticks, diced
250g (9oz) chestnut mushrooms, finely sliced
3 tablespoons tamari or soy sauce
¼–½ hot chilli, finely chopped, or chilli flakes, added to taste
1 large turnip, or ¼ daikon or a handful of radishes, cubed or sliced
400g (14oz) konjac noodles
a large handful of baby spinach leaves

Per serving 17g carbs, 2.3g fibre, 7.1g protein, 1.2g fat, 107kcal

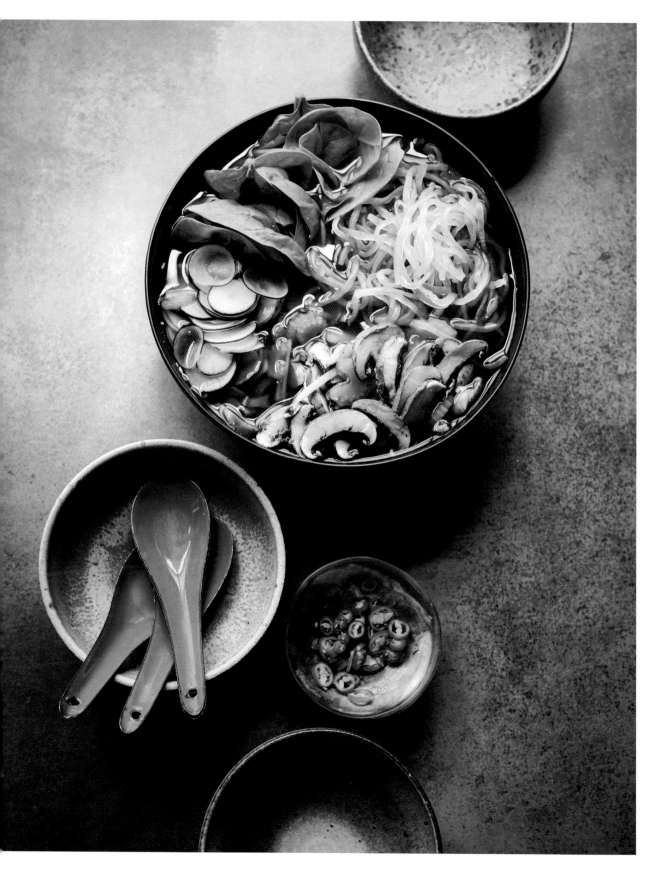

Salmon, Lemon & Parsley Pâté

Red lentils are a comforting contrast to the flaky, oily fish and the sharp, zesty lemon. They also provide fibre and satiety, and help the fish go further, making this pâté economical as well as tasty. Any salmon will work here, from tinned red salmon, hot smoked, fresh or shreds of the finest smoked salmon, each bringing a different taste and texture. Accompany it with the Flaxseed Crackers (opposite), the Flaxseed Bread Rolls (page 101), a boiled egg and hunks of cucumber and tomatoes. You can see a jar of pâté on page 104.

Wash and drain the lentils. Put them into a saucepan and fill with cold water. Bring to the boil and add a good pinch of salt. Reduce the heat, skim any scum off the surface and cook for 15–20 minutes, but do check the packet instructions; some lentils take more or less time. Drain and leave to cool.

Meanwhile, if the salmon isn't already cooked, roast it for about 20 minutes in a preheated oven at 200°C/180°C fan/400°F/gas mark 6. Let it cool.

Remove any skin or bones from the salmon and flake it into a bowl. Add the remaining ingredients. Mix gently so that the pâté still has some texture. Season to taste with salt and pepper and a little more lemon zest, if it needs it. Transfer it into an airtight container and keep in the fridge for up to 3 days.

SERVES 6

100g (3½oz) dried red lentils
180g–200g (6–7oz) hot-smoked or fresh salmon
1 teaspoon lemon zest, or more to taste
juice of 1 lemon
10g (¼oz) parsley, roughly chopped
125g (4½oz) full-fat soft cheese
salt and freshly ground black pepper

Per serving 3.8g carbs, 0.7g fibre, 11g protein, 8.1g fat, 134kcal

Flaxseed Crackers

These versatile crackers are perfect for accompanying a dip, taking to work or making a healthier version of nachos (see page 138). Try flavouring the crackers with dried herbs, such as rosemary, thyme or oregano, or seeds, such as black onion, cumin or caraway or make the Spicy Tortilla Chip flavour below.

Preheat the oven to 180°C/160°C fan/350°F/gas mark 4. Line two baking trays with baking parchment and brush them generously with oil.

Whizz all the ingredients together, including the flavourings if making spicy tortilla chips, in a food processor by blitzing briefly until all of the seeds are a little broken up. Leave the mixture for 10 minutes and stir. As the seeds absorb the moisture, you should be left with a rough, thick paste that is spreadable but still has a little texture to it.

Use a spatula to divide the mixture between the two trays.

Take a piece of baking parchment the size of your baking trays and brush it generously with oil. Place it, oiled side down, on top of the mixture on the first tray and spread it out with your hands so that the cracker mixture is even and about 2mm (1/16in) thick. It should form a rectangle that almost fills the tray. Peel off the paper and use it to do the same with the second tray.

Neaten the edges with a spatula and cook for 15–18 minutes or until the edges become golden brown. Remove the trays from the oven. Slide the crackers on the paper onto a chopping board. Now either break the crackers into shards or use a sharp knife to cut them into squares, rectangles or triangles as you wish. Loosen them from the paper and spread them out over the trays, without the paper. Put them back into the oven for a further 5–10 minutes or until they are dry and lightly browned.

Once they are bone-dry, the crackers will keep in an airtight container for a week. If they soften, re-bake them in a hot oven for a few minutes.

SERVES 12

extra virgin olive oil, to grease
150g (5½oz) mixed seeds made up of sunflower, pumpkin, poppy, hemp, coriander or sesame
50g (1¾oz) milled flaxseed
1 teaspoon salt
1 egg
25g (1oz) gram (chickpea) flour
200ml (7fl oz) water

For Spicy Tortilla Chips

1 heaped teaspoon smoked paprika
1 heaped teaspoon garlic powder
1 teaspoon cayenne pepper

Per serving 3.7g carbs, 1.9g fibre, 5.6g protein, 9.8g fat, 130kcal

Amal's Spinach Falafel & Beetroot Hummus

Amal Alquatani is a good friend of ours from Kuwait. She loves to cook for parties and large family gatherings. Any leftovers are perfect to take to work the next day. Here she uses half spinach and half chickpeas in the recipe to reduce the carb count. One standard can will do for the falafel and the hummus. I use frozen spinach to make these; it doesn't need to be cooked, but do make sure it is defrosted and squeezed very dry before using.

Preheat the oven to 200°C/180°C fan/400°F/gas mark 6. Put the sesame seeds in a bowl. Put everything else in the food processor and pulse the mixture to a bumpy paste. Grease a baking tray with a little olive oil.

Roll the mixture into 20 walnut-size balls using your hands and drop into the sesame seeds to coat. Press them into shape – you want them about 5cm (2in) in diameter. Put them onto the baking tray and make a shallow hole in the top of each one with your finger. Cook for 30 minutes or until lightly browned. Serve warm or at room temperature with the hummus.

MAKES 20 FALAFEL

50g (1¾oz) sesame seeds, to coat
1 small leek, finely chopped
1 small brown onion, roughly chopped
2 garlic cloves, finely chopped
25g (1oz) coriander, finely chopped
150g (5½oz) very well squeezed cooked spinach (or use frozen, defrosted from approx. 500g/1lb 2oz weight)
50g (1¾oz) ground almonds
120g (4¼oz) cooked chickpeas (½ x 400g/14oz can), well drained
1 teaspoon ground cumin
1 teaspoon salt
½ teaspoon chilli flakes
a generous amount of freshly ground black pepper
50g (1¾oz) sesame seeds, to coat
olive oil, to grease

Per falafel 1.7g carbs, 1.1g fibre, 2.1g protein, 3.1g fat, 45kcal
Per serving of beetroot hummus 5.1g carbs, 1.6g fibre, 4.4g protein, 9.8g fat, 130kcal

Beetroot hummus

This happy pink dip is wonderful in contrast to green falafel or the fresh green herbs and salad often served with it. Enjoy it with cold chicken, the Chicken Shawarma (page 132), low-carb crackers or bread (see pages 85 and 101).

SERVES 8

1 medium raw or cooked beetroot (weighing approx. 125g/ 4¼oz)
2 tablespoons olive oil
3 tablespoons tahini
120g (4¼oz) chickpeas (½ x 400g/14oz can), well drained
juice of ½ lemon
4 tablespoons Greek yogurt
salt and freshly ground black pepper

Boil the raw beetroot for 45 minutes– 1 hour until tender, then drain. If you are using cooked, omit this step. Put all the ingredients except the yogurt in a food processor and blitz until smooth. Stir in the yogurt, then adjust the seasoning to taste. The dip will keep in the fridge for up to 5 days.

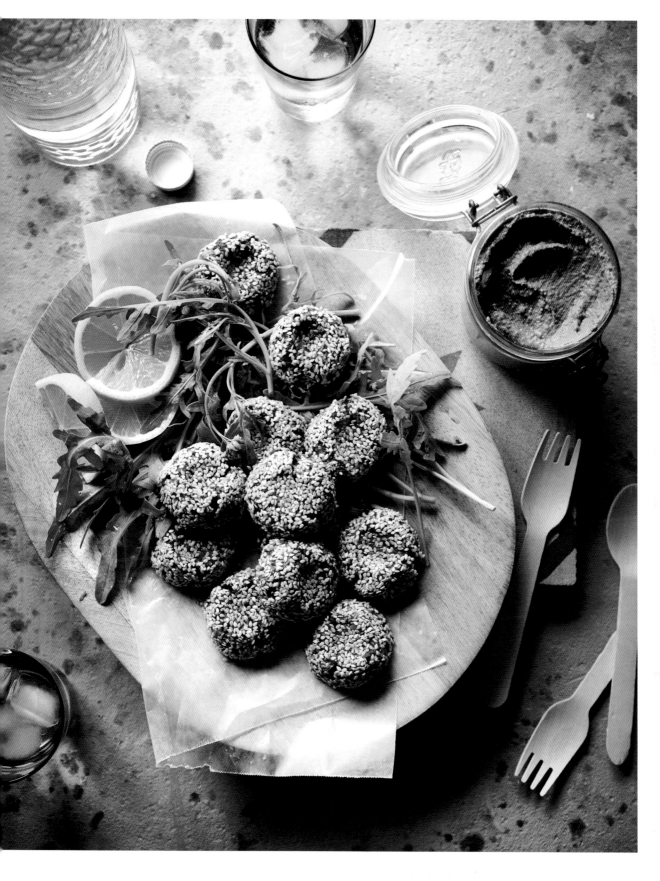

Italian Seafood Salad

This is my cheat's Italian seafood salad with a little British smoked salmon thrown in for colour and extra flavour. If you are lucky enough to have a good fishmonger near you, do use freshly cooked seafood. I live miles from the sea, so I buy bags of frozen cooked seafood, which I defrost overnight in the fridge. What the frozen version lacks in flavour it makes up for with convenience, but I do urge you to taste the dressing to make sure it is punchy and balanced with seasoning. If you are going to pack this up for work or a picnic, invest in an insulated lunchbox or keep the container cool with an ice-pack until you can eat it, or store it in the fridge at work.

Mix all the ingredients together in a large mixing bowl. Allow the flavours to mingle for 5 minutes and then taste and adjust the seasoning and acidity as necessary. Serve chilled with low-carb bread (see pages 101 and 124) to mop up the delicious oil and juices.

SERVES 4

350g (12oz) cooked seafood, such as prawns, clams, mussels and squid
2 celery sticks, finely sliced
1 small carrot, julienned
1 tablespoon small capers, washed and drained
¼–½ red chilli, finely chopped, or a pinch of chilli flakes
50g (1¾oz) smoked salmon, roughly torn
1 tablespoon lemon juice, or more as necessary
1 tablespoon white wine vinegar, or more as necessary
4 tablespoons extra virgin olive oil
2 tablespoons flat-leaf parsley
6 sun-dried tomatoes, roughly chopped (optional)
½ teaspoon salt
plenty of freshly ground black pepper

Per serving 6.2g carbs, 1.7g fibre, 17g protein, 21g fat, 282kcal

Quick-fried Paprika Spiced Chicken, Avocado & Lemon Yogurt Dressing

This is lovely to take on a picnic or to pack up and take to work. Cook the chicken the night before and let it cool to room temperature before storing in the fridge. Put the dressing in a small jar and take the zested lemon with it to squeeze over the salad and chicken.

Mix the paprika, cumin and pepper on a medium plate. Season the chicken with salt, then roll in the powdered spice on the plate. Heat the oil in a non-stick frying pan over a medium heat until hot. Fry the chicken on both sides for 10–15 minutes or until cooked through and no longer pink inside.

Meanwhile, make the dressing. Mix together the yogurt, lemon zest and olive oil in a bowl and season to taste. This will keep in the fridge, covered, for 3 days.

Serve the chicken warm from the pan if you are enjoying at home or cold with the dressing, avocado, salad leaves and herbs, cherry tomatoes and lemon wedges from the grated lemon for squeezing over the top.

SERVES 2

1 tablespoon smoked paprika
1 teaspoon ground cumin
½ teaspoon freshly ground black pepper
6 mini chicken fillets or 250g (9oz) boneless, skinless chicken breast, cut into finger-width slices
2 tablespoons extra virgin olive oil
1 avocado, sliced
a handful of salad leaves
a few sprigs of herbs, such as basil, parsley or coriander
6 cherry tomatoes
salt
lemon wedges, to serve

For the lemon yogurt dressing
4 tablespoons thick Greek yogurt
1 teaspoon finely grated lemon zest
2 teaspoons extra virgin olive oil
salt and freshly ground black pepper

Per serving 7.6g carbs, 3.5g fibre, 37g protein, 28g fat, 442kcal

Vietnamese Chicken Salad

On our travels to Vietnam, I was amazed to see the quantity of herbs used, huge bunches of them, instead of salad leaves. They give so much zing and flavour; don't stint on them. If you don't have enough of one herb, just add more of another.

If you use red cabbage, your chicken will be purple in colour, which is amusing although the flavour is the same. This recipe is a good way to use up leftover cooked chicken or turkey, in which case miss out the poaching instructions. Traditionally, the dressing has garlic, but you can omit this if you care about breathing over colleagues!

Soak the spring onions in cold water for 15 minutes, then drain and set aside. Poach the chicken in a saucepan of boiling salted water for 15–20 minutes or until cooked through and no longer pink inside. Leave to cool in the water for 10 minutes, then drain and leave to cool completely.

Toast the sesame seeds in a dry pan, stirring frequently until they start to pop and turn golden brown, then remove from the heat and tip onto a plate to cool.

Mix the dressing ingredients together in a small bowl.

Finely slice the cabbage with a very sharp knife on a chopping board. Take time to get the shreds very thinly sliced. Tear the chicken into shreds. Cut the carrot and pepper with a sharp knife into julienne strips, or use a gadget that shreds, and add them straight into the dressing in a large bowl to prevent them browning.

To assemble the salad, mix the chicken, cabbage, peanuts and herbs into the bowl with the carrot, pepper, ginger and dressing. Arrange on a serving platter and scatter over the toasted sesame seeds.

SERVES 2

3 spring onions, finely sliced
2 boneless, skinless chicken breasts
2 tablespoons sesame seeds
150g (5½oz) white or red cabbage
1 small carrot
½ red or yellow pepper
50g (1¾oz) roasted peanuts
a large handful of a mixture of Thai basil, coriander and mint, leaves roughly torn and stalks finely chopped
1 tablespoon finely grated ginger

For the dressing

juice of 2 limes
4 tablespoons Vietnamese fish sauce or 3 tablespoons nam pla
3 tablespoons rice vinegar
1 teaspoon mild honey
¼–½ hot red or green chilli, finely chopped or a good pinch of chilli flakes
1 small garlic clove, finely chopped or grated (optional)

Per serving 20g carbs, 8g fibre, 41g protein, 27g fat, 522kcal

Food on the Go Tip

To make this portable, mix the salad minus the herbs with the dressing and pack into a jar or sealable box. Put the herbs on top so that they don't wilt, and mix when you eat it. It will keep chilled like this for 2 days.

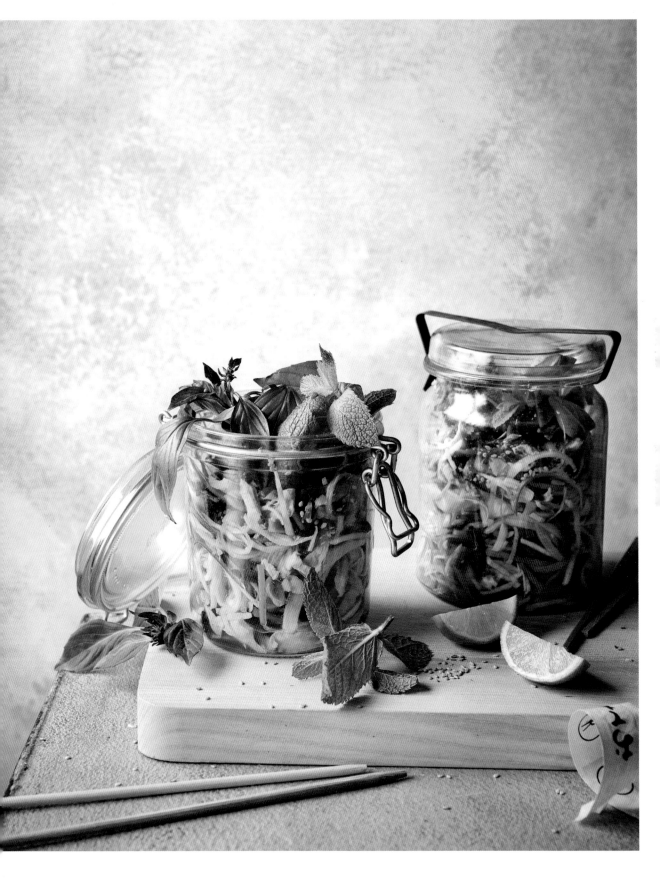

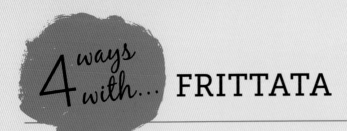

4 ways with... FRITTATA

There was a time when our publishers cried out "No more frittata!", as I was constantly writing Italian cookbooks and had become obsessed with the ubiquitous eggy invention. In defence of the humble frittata, they are easy, economical, versatile and, moreover, tasty. Here I have been allowed to roam through frittata recipes, pick out my top four and discover the best way to cook them. In Italy they are made on the hob in a frying pan, but there is the problem of flipping them over, which can be humiliating and messy. You can finish them under the grill in the pan but you have a hot handle, which I forget not to touch. For me, the way forward with a fuss-free frittata is to bake it.

Oven-baked Individual Frittata

Individual frittatas are easy to knock up and take to work or can be made for a hot breakfast while you take a shower. What you put in them is up to you, from fresh herbs to yesterday's leftover cooked vegetables, meat and fish.

Preheat the oven to 200°C/180°C fan/400°F/gas mark 6.

Generously butter a ramekin 8 x 4cm (3¼ x 1½in) and put a circle of baking parchment at the bottom (please don't bother with scissors and a compass, a roughly torn piece of baking parchment is fine).

Beat the egg with seasoning and stir in the additional ingredients. Pour the mixture into the ramekin and bake for 12–15 minutes or until cooked through. Allow the frittata to cool for a few minutes before turning out and eating or let it cool to room temperature before packing up in a lunchbox. The frittata will keep in the fridge for 2 days, so do make a batch.

MAKES 1 FRITATTA
butter, to grease
1 egg
50g (1¾oz) leftovers, such as cooked vegetables, cooked meat, fish or Italian Roast Vegetables (page 68)
a small handful of herbs, such as basil, thyme or oregano, roughly torn
10g (¼oz) cheese, grated (optional)
salt and freshly ground black pepper

Per serving 5.7g carbs, 3.1g fibre, 12g protein, 12g fat, 186kcal

Microwave Mug Frittata

I prefer to eat these while they are still warm, so they are ideal for breakfast or a light meal. They are so easy and quick to make that you could prepare them at work if you have a microwave. Pack up the egg, a block of cheese, cooked meat and herbs and off you go, equipped to make a satisfying hot meal for lunch.

Beat the egg with seasoning in a microwaveable mug. Stir in the rest of the ingredients and microwave for 1 minute and 30 seconds on high or until cooked through. Remove the mug and invert it onto a plate. Let the frittata cool for a few minutes before eating.

SERVES 1
1 egg
50g (1½oz) cooked meat and vegetables
10g (¼oz) Cheddar or other hard cheese, cubed
a few leaves of coriander, parsley or basil, roughly torn
salt and freshly ground black pepper

Per serving 5.7g carbs, 3.1g fibre, 12g protein, 12g fat, 186kcal

Oven-baked Greek Frittata

This has all the flavour of a Greek cheese pie with none of the carb-heavy pastry and a slice is ideal to take to work.

Preheat the oven to 200°C/180°C fan/400°F/gas mark 6. Line a baking tray with baking parchment or a silicone mat. Line an ovenproof dish measuring roughly 25 x 20 x 6cm (10 x 8 x 2½in) with baking parchment. The easiest way to do this is to run the paper under the tap and scrunch it into a ball. Spread it out and shake off the excess water. It will become soft and you can push it into the dish more easily.

Spread the courgette on the lined baking tray. Brush with 1 tablespoon of the olive oil and cook for 10 minutes. Remove from the oven and set aside.

Meanwhile, fry the leek in the remaining oil and the butter in a frying pan over a medium heat. Season in the pan. It will take about 10 minutes to soften. When tender, set aside to cool.

Beat the eggs in a large mixing bowl. Crumble in the feta and stir in the remaining ingredients. Pour into the prepared dish and bake for 25–30 minutes or until it is firm to the touch. Remove from the oven and leave to cool for 10 minutes before serving.

SERVES 6

1 large courgette, approx. 200g (7oz), finely sliced
3 tablespoons extra virgin olive oil
1 leek or 6 spring onions, finely sliced
a knob of butter
8 eggs
200g (7oz) feta
25g (1oz) Parmesan or Grana Padano, finely grated
150g (5½oz) cooked and squeezed spinach, roughly chopped (400g/14oz frozen weight)
10g (¼oz) dill, finely chopped
salt and freshly ground black pepper

Per serving 1.6g carbs, 2.9g fibre, 18g protein, 23g fat, 288kcal

Layered Tuna & Pepper Frittata

For such a simple mix of ingredients, this frittata has knock-out flavour. Serve warm or cool and slice for a packed lunch.

Preheat the oven to 200°C/180°C fan/400°F/gas mark 6. Fry the onions in the oil in a frying pan over a low heat. They will take about 15 minutes to soften. Season in the pan.

Meanwhile, line an ovenproof dish roughly 25 x 20 x 6cm (10 x 8 x 2½in) with baking parchment (see above).

Beat the eggs in a bowl with seasoning.

Spoon the onions into the prepared dish. Pour over roughly one-third of the beaten egg. Lay the peppers over the onions, add another third of the egg and scatter over the drained tuna. Pour over the remaining egg and top with the cheese, if using.

Bake for 30–35 minutes or until cooked through and lightly browned on top.

SERVES 6

2 brown onions, sliced into rings
3 tablespoons extra virgin olive oil
8 eggs
150g (5½oz) roasted red peppers in oil, drained on kitchen paper
2 x 250g (7oz) cans of tuna in oil or water, drained
25g (1oz) Parmesan, finely grated (optional)
salt and freshly ground black pepper

Per serving 4.3g carbs, 2.6g fibre, 21g protein, 17g fat, 258kcal

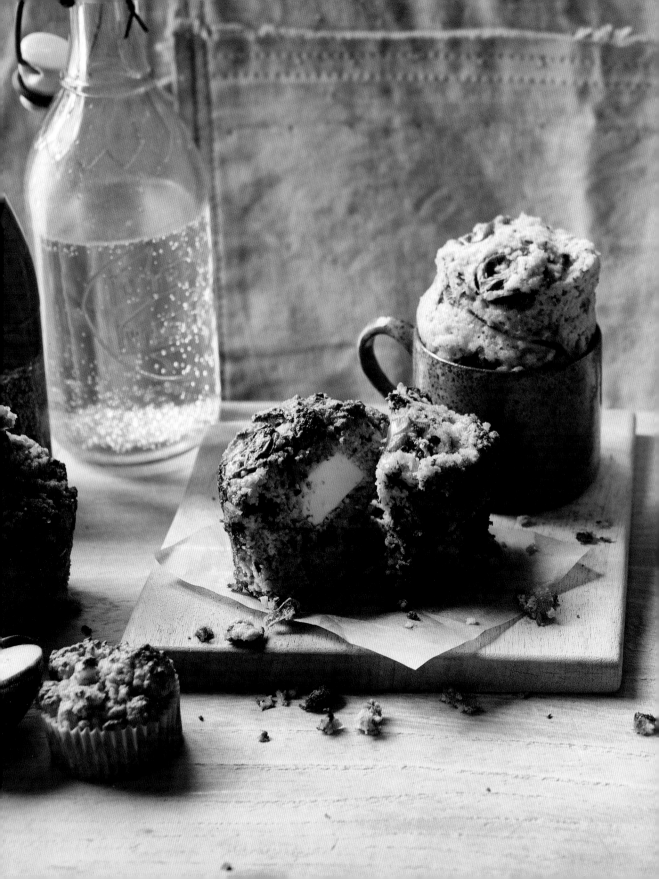

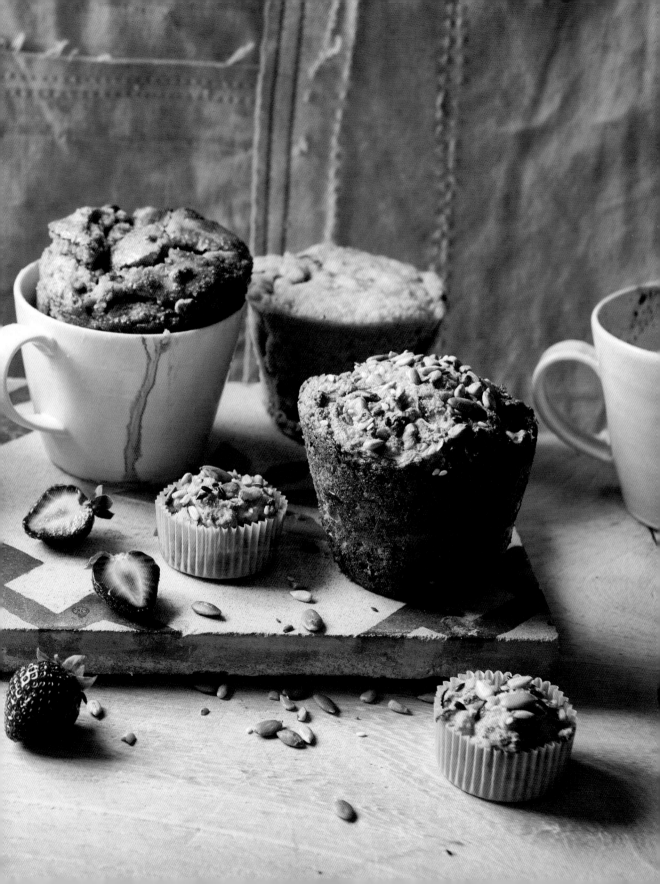

MAGIC MUFFINS

These were so popular from *The Diabetes Weight-loss Cookbook* that we have come up with more ways to cook them for this book. The muffins are an adaptation of the popular mug cake, but with a fraction of the carbs. It's a really versatile basic recipe that can be adapted to sweet and savoury flavours.

Basic Magic Muffin

These muffins can be made sweet with an apple or savoury with a courgette. The mixture can make one large mug muffin, two smaller ones or 12 mini muffins. It's such a versatile basic recipe that can be adapted to sweet and savoury flavours.

Mix the egg and fat together in a bowl. Add the ground almonds, baking powder, the grated fruit or courgette and either the vanilla extract and spice (for a sweet version) or seasoning (for a savoury version) and mix well. Spoon the mixture into one or two microwaveable mugs. Microwave on full power for 2½ minutes or until cooked through.

Alternatively, to cook them in the oven, generously grease and line the mugs or use paper-lined or silicone muffin moulds. Preheat the oven to 200°C/180°C fan/400°F/gas mark 6 and bake for 20–25 minutes. You can also divide the mixture between 12 mini muffin cases and bake for 10–12 minutes. Check the muffins are cooked through by piercing them with a skewer. If it comes out clean, they are done; if it is wet, put them back into the oven for another few minutes.

SERVES 1–2/Makes 1 standard-size mug muffin

1 egg
a knob of butter, melted, or
* 2 teaspoons coconut or olive oil*
50g (1¾oz) ground almonds
½ teaspoon baking powder
½ apple or pear or ½ medium
* courgette, coarsely grated*
½ teaspoon vanilla extract and/
* or pinch of ground cinnamon or*
* mixed spice (for sweet muffins)*
salt and freshly ground black pepper
* (for savoury muffins)*

Per apple muffin 13g carbs, 8.3g fibre, 20g protein, 42g fat, 526kcal
Per courgette muffin 5.1g carbs, 9.4g fibre, 21g protein, 42g fat, 500kcal

Pink Berry Mug Muffin

This fun pink-coloured muffin is naturally sweet and ideal cut into circles and topped with cream and berries.

Cut half the strawberries into small pieces and put them into a bowl. Mush them to a pulp with a fork. Mix with the remaining ingredients and spoon into a mug. Cook as in the recipe for Basic Magic Muffin above.

SERVES 1–2/Makes 1 standard-size mug muffin

70g (2½oz) strawberries, hulled
1 egg
a knob of butter, melted, or
* 2 teaspoons coconut oil*
50g (1¾oz) ground almonds
½ teaspoon baking powder

Per muffin 7.9g carbs, 10g fibre, 20g protein, 42g fat, 508kcal

Anna's Greek Feta Mug Muffins

Our friend Anna Hudson came up with this idea for a wonderful treat to take to work or on picnics. They taste delicious and you have everything you need for a satisfying lunch. They are quite filling, so we have divided the mixture into two. You can make them in small mugs or cups in the microwave as well as in the oven if you grease and line cups, or use silicone muffin moulds. They are great on their own or serve them with soup.

Mix the egg, butter, almonds, tomatoes, courgette, baking powder, seasoning and oregano together in a bowl. Spoon half of the mixture into two small microwaveable mugs. Tuck pieces of feta into the centre of the mugs and cover with the remaining mixture. Arrange the halved tomatoes onto the tops, cut side up. Cook as for the Basic Magic Muffin (opposite).

SERVES 2/Makes 2 small mug muffins

1 egg
a knob of butter, melted, or 2 teaspoons olive oil
50g (1¾oz) ground almonds
1 tablespoon chopped sun-dried or fresh tomatoes
½ courgette, coarsely grated
½ teaspoon baking powder
1 teaspoon dried oregano
2 x 15g (½oz) cubes of feta
5 cherry tomatoes, halved
salt and freshly ground black pepper

Per muffin 4.1g carbs, 5.2g fibre, 13g protein, 24g fat, 299kcal

Nutty Seeded Muffins

This simple muffin is an ideal low-carb substitute for a wholemeal seeded roll. It is the perfect match for butter and cheese, smoked salmon and cream cheese, or for toasting in slices and enjoying with butter and Marmite. It is filling, so is ideal split into two portions.

Mix all the ingredients together as in the Basic Magic Muffin recipe (opposite) and follow the cooking instructions. Experiment with the flavour variations suggested below.

Makes 1 standard-size mug muffin

1 egg
½ courgette, coarsely grated
50g (1¾oz) ground almonds
½ teaspoon baking powder
1 tablespoon mixed seeds
a pinch of salt and plenty of freshly ground black pepper
1 tablespoon finely chopped sun-dried tomatoes, plus a teaspoon of the oil from the jar
6 walnut halves, roughly chopped

Per muffin 8.4g carbs, 12g fibre, 25g protein, 55g fat, 651kcal

Variations

- 1 teaspoon black onion seeds
- 15g (½oz) Parmesan or Grana Padano, finely grated
- a pinch of chilli flakes

Spicy Nuts & Crispy Kale

If I leave a jar of these out at home they will be gone in minutes, but at least I know my family aren't diving into fried corn or potato crisps that will shoot their blood glucose levels up, then bring them crashing down again. These are great for entertaining, taking to work or filling up hungry children.

Preheat the oven to 200°C/180°C fan/400°F/gas mark 6.

Toss the nuts and seeds in a bowl with 1 tablespoon of the oil, the chilli flakes, ground ginger and 1 tablespoon of the soy sauce. Pour onto a baking tray and flatten them out into a single layer. Roast for 5 minutes.

Meanwhile, toss the kale in the bowl with the remaining oil and soy sauce and then add it to the tray. Roast for a further 3–5 minutes or until lightly browned and crisp. Allow to cool to room temperature and serve. The mixture will keep well in an airtight container for up to a week (kept out of sight of hungry teenagers).

SERVES 6

200g (7oz) mixed nuts, such as pecans, almonds, walnuts and macadamia nuts
2 tablespoons sesame seeds
2 tablespoons toasted sesame oil
½ teaspoon chilli flakes
1 teaspoon ground ginger
2 tablespoons soy sauce
100g kale or cavolo nero, tough stems removed, torn into 5cm (2in) pieces

Per serving 4g carbs, 3.7g fibre, 7.2g protein, 26g fat, 288kcal

Spiced Chicken Liver Pâté

This is a wonderful Middle Eastern way to serve livers; a sort of rough-ish pâté to spoon onto any of the low-carb breads on pages 101 and 124. It is normally served as part of a mezze by our Kuwaiti friend Amal, but it is good too as a lunch to take to work or a starter.

Heat the oil in a large frying pan and fry the onion, chilli, garlic, the salt and some pepper for about 5 minutes or until soft. Roughly chop the chicken or lamb's livers into bite-size pieces (I do this with a pair of scissors while the livers are still in their container) and add to the pan with the cumin and turmeric to taste. Cook for 10–15 minutes, stirring frequently, over a medium heat or until the livers are no longer pink inside and cooked through. Add the pomegranate molasses and lemon juice towards end of cooking. Taste and adjust the seasoning as necessary.

Serve warm or at room temperature. The dish will keep, covered, in the fridge for up to 4 days.

SERVES 6 (AS PART OF A MEZZE)

4 tablespoons extra virgin olive oil
1 medium white or red onion, finely sliced
¼–½ hot red or green chilli, finely chopped
2 garlic cloves, finely chopped
400g (14oz) chicken or lamb's livers
½ teaspoon ground cumin
½ teaspoon ground turmeric
2 teaspoons pomegranate molasses
1 tablespoon lemon juice
½ teaspoon salt
freshly ground black pepper

Per serving 4.6g carbs, 0.7g fibre, 10g protein, 11g fat, 164kcal

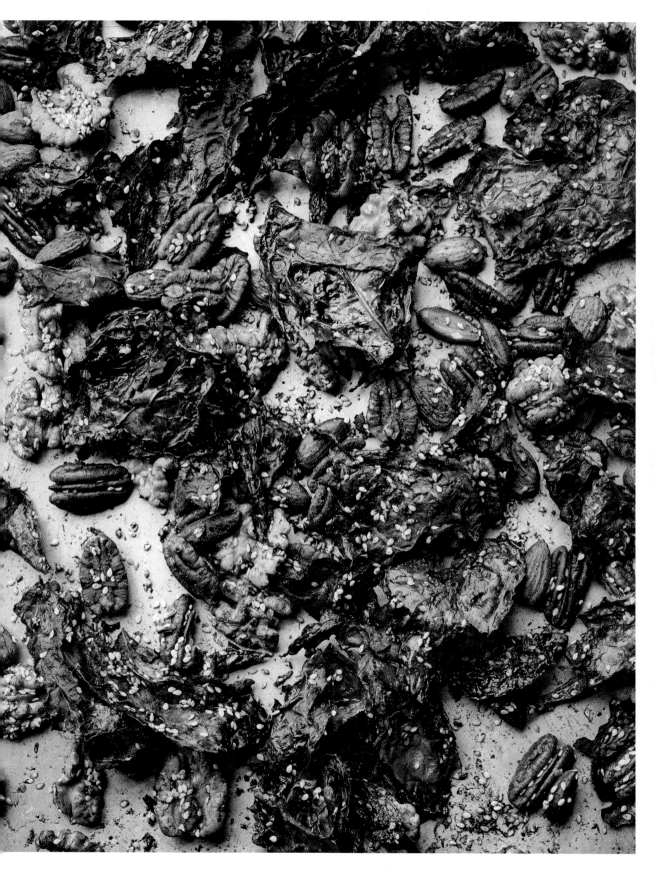

Spinach Sheets for Wraps & Pasta

I invented this recipe for our previous book so that Giancarlo could eat his favourite lasagne without the gluten and a huge carb load. If you imagine a thin but strong spinach omelette, you will have got the gist of these versatile, light sheets. In this book they are used for wraps to take to work (see page 102) and cannelloni (see page 146).

We usually use frozen roughly chopped spinach for this. It is sold in 900g–1kg (2–2¼lb) bags and, to give you a guide, 900g (2lb) of frozen spinach becomes about 300g (10½oz) once it is defrosted and squeezed well. Don't buy finely chopped spinach if you have the choice as it is harder to squeeze dry.

Preheat the oven to 220°C/200°C fan/425°F/gas mark 7. Line two baking trays with baking parchment and grease with the olive oil.

Blitz all the ingredients in a food processor to form a paste. Divide the mixture between the lined trays. Put another piece of oiled baking parchment over the top and carefully press it out to form thin rectangles measuring roughly 27 x 34cm (10¾ x 13½in) and about 5mm (¼in) thick. Don't worry if they are slightly less than this. Remove the top sheet of paper. Tidy it up as necessary and even it out with a flat-ended tool, such as a fish slice or dough scraper.

Bake for 8–10 minutes or until the sheets are firm to the touch and set through. Remove from the oven and leave to cool on the tray.

After cooking the sheets can be cut into any shapes or sizes you like. They can be rolled around oiled baking parchment and covered with clingfilm and either kept refrigerated for up to 3 days or frozen for 3 months.

MAKES:
2 sheets of pasta approx. 36 x 30cm (14¼ x 12in)
or 18 rectangles measuring approx. 10 x 12cm (4 x 4½in) for the cannelloni (page 146)
or 12 wraps 15 x 9cm (6 x 3½in)

extra virgin olive oil, to grease
approx. 300g (10½oz) defrosted spinach, squeezed dry from a 900g (2lb) bag of frozen spinach
½ teaspoon salt
4 eggs
8 tablespoons nut or cow's milk
1 heaped tablespoon psyllium husk powder

Per wrap 0.5g carbs, 2.5g fibre, 6.2g protein, 4g fat, 68kcal

Flaxseed Bread Rolls

Golden flaxseed (linseed) is easy to buy in supermarkets and online. It can be ground to a sand-like texture in a food processor and gives a nutty, dense texture similar to wholemeal brown bread. Brown flaxseed is often sold ready ground and will work fine, but the colour of the bread will be darker and the texture may vary. Flaxseed does become rancid over time, so it is better kept in the fridge or freezer.

Preheat the oven to 200°C/180°C fan/400°F/gas mark 6. Line a baking tray with a silicone mat or baking parchment.

Use a large metal spoon to mix all the dry ingredients together in a large mixing bowl. Stir in the eggs, water and any flavouring suggestions. Once you have a well-combined dough, relax for 10 minutes and let the dough do the same. During that time the flaxseed will absorb the water. Use your hands to gather it into a ball and remove it from the bowl.

Divide the dough into four and, using lightly wetted hands, roll each piece into a ball. Put them on the lined baking tray, spaced at least 4cm (1½in) apart. Flatten and shape them into rounds about 9cm (3½in) diameter. Bake for 20 minutes or until the rolls are lightly browned and firm to the touch. Remove from the oven and allow to cool on a wire rack before slicing and filling. Mini rolls should measure 4cm (1½in) across and will take about 15 minutes to cook. The rolls are best kept in the fridge in a container for up to 4 days or frozen for up to 3 months.

MAKES 4 LARGE ROLLS OR 12 MINI ROLLS
150g (5½oz) ground flaxseed
1 teaspoon baking powder
1 teaspoon salt
2 eggs, beaten
50ml (2fl oz) cold water

Optional flavourings
100g (3½oz) walnuts, roughly chopped
50g (1¾oz) sunflower seeds
2 teaspoons caraway seeds
1 teaspoon dried oregano
25g (1oz) Parmesan, finely grated

Per large roll 0.6g carbs, 11g fibre, 12g protein, 20g fat, 251kcal
Per small roll 0g carbs, 3.8g fibre, 3.9g protein, 6.6g fat, 84kcal

Variation Rosemary & Olive Rolls

This makes a good bread to dip into balsamic and olive oil and serve with drinks or it's delicious to mop up the juices from the Prawn & Chorizo Traybake on page 72, with one of the soups from chapter 1, or to take to work with any of the dips and filling ideas on page 106.

MAKES 8 SMALL ROLLS
2 teaspoons finely chopped rosemary, plus a little to sprinkle
16 green or black olives, pitted and roughly chopped
salt flakes
extra virgin olive oil, to drizzle

Follow the recipe above, adding the herbs and olives with the water, and mix thoroughly. Divide the dough into 8 small balls, flatten and shape, and top each one with a few rosemary needles and salt flakes. Bake for 15 minutes or until cooked through. Cool on a wire rack drizzled with a little olive oil.

Spinach Wraps, Carrot & Walnut Salad & Tahini Yogurt

Who needs the carbs from a flour wrap when you can have a zero-carb homemade spinach one instead? The tahini yogurt is perfect to hold the wrap and salad in place. You could also use the One-minute Mayonnaise (page 78) with some shredded ham hock or the Horseradish & Lemon Crème Fraîche (page 74) with salmon flakes.

To make the salad, put the onion into cold water for about 10 minutes to remove its strength. Put the carrots into a mixing bowl with the lemon juice to stop them going brown. Add the walnuts, celery, nigella seeds, oil and the drained onion and stir through. Season to taste and serve straight away or keep it in the fridge for a couple of days.

To make up the wraps, generously spread the tahini yogurt onto the wrap. Add a few spoons of the carrot and walnut salad, roll up the wrap into a spiral and you are ready to go.

SERVES 2

1 fat spring onion, finely sliced
200g (7oz) carrots, coarsely grated
juice of ½ lemon
50g (2oz) walnuts, roughly chopped
1 celery stick, finely sliced
½ teaspoon nigella seeds
2 tablespoons extra virgin olive oil
4 spinach wraps (page 100)
salt and freshly ground black pepper

Per serving of salad 9.5g carbs, 6g fibre, 5.1g protein, 30g fat, 342kcal
Per serving of tahini yogurt 3.6g carbs, 1.5g fibre, 7.9g protein, 30g fat, 322kcal
Per wrap 0.5g carbs, 2.5g fibre, 6.2g protein, 4g fat, 68kcal

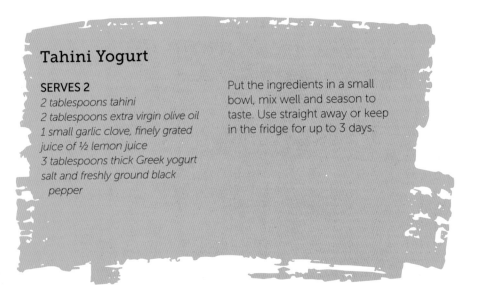

Tahini Yogurt

SERVES 2
2 tablespoons tahini
2 tablespoons extra virgin olive oil
1 small garlic clove, finely grated
juice of ½ lemon juice
3 tablespoons thick Greek yogurt
salt and freshly ground black pepper

Put the ingredients in a small bowl, mix well and season to taste. Use straight away or keep in the fridge for up to 3 days.

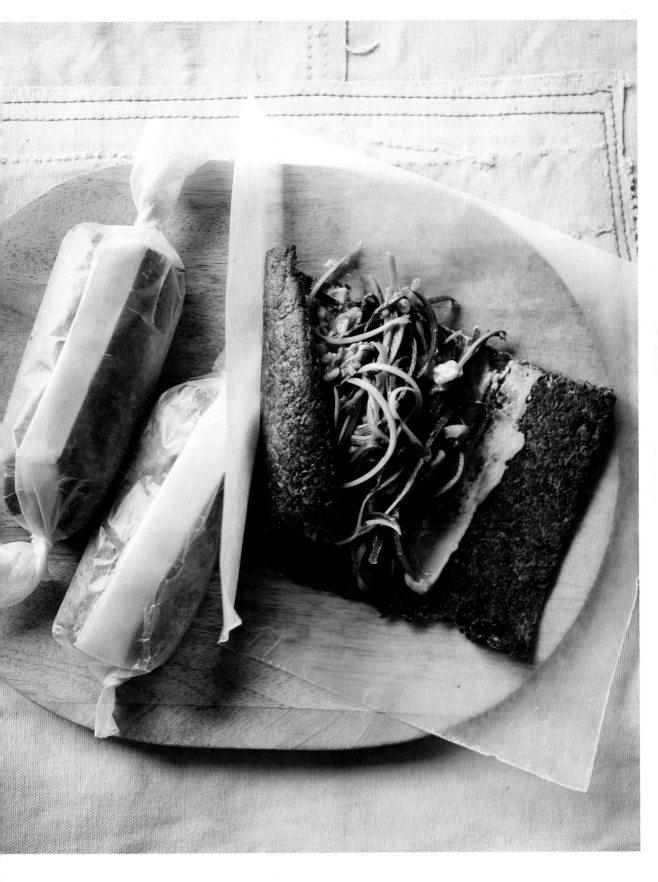

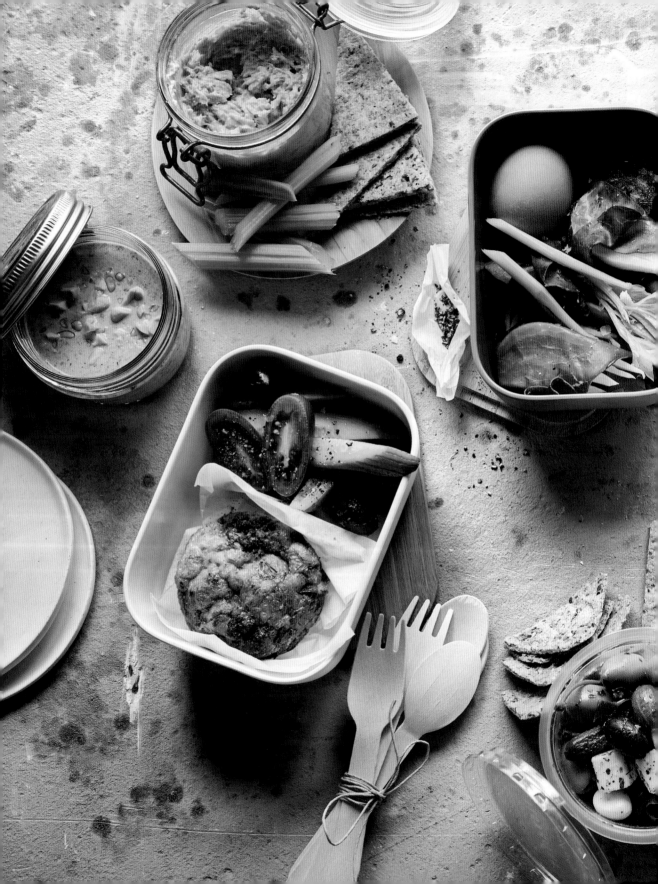

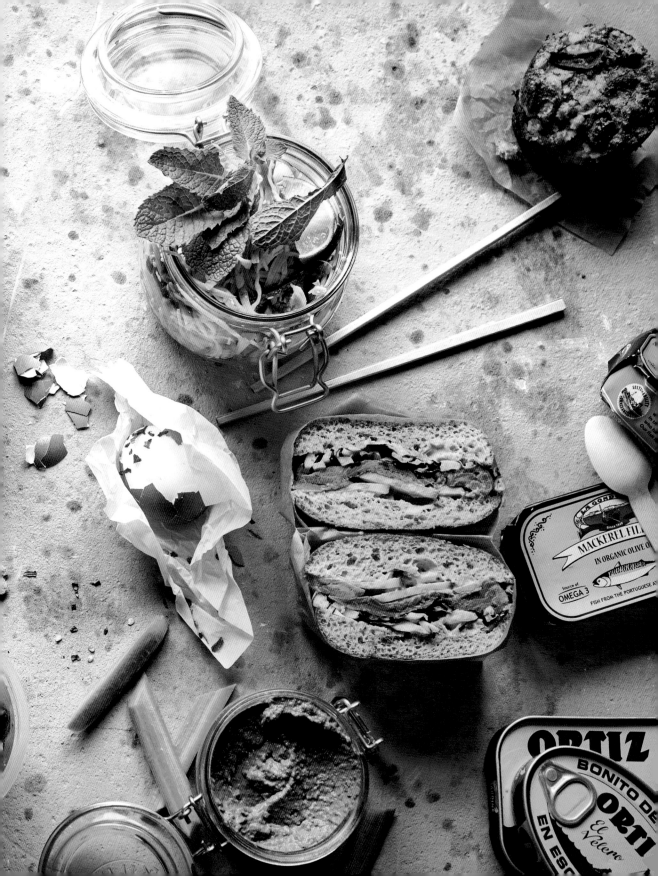

Simple Lunch Ideas

1 Be prepared! This is our motto so that temptation doesn't get the better of us when we are hungry and away from home. Dr Unwin carries a ring-pull tin of sardines in his car and a teaspoon! Giancarlo has walnuts in his. I have a few pecans and two squares of dark chocolate in my handbag. Jenny frequently takes a pot of apple wedges with mixed nuts and cinnamon out with her and Jen has pork scratchings (with no sugar or additives).

2 Other ideas to pick up and carry are boiled eggs – crack them as soon as they are boiled to stop the blue ring appearing around the yolk, but leave them in the shell. Wrap them in a piece of baking parchment with salt or celery salt and pepper ready for dipping.

3 Buy sliced beef, chicken or ham and use them as wraps for avocado, lettuce, our Peri-peri Dipping Sauce (page 112), mayo and lemon – just watch the ingredients for added sugar, flavourings and preservatives.

4 Sticks of Cheddar, tomatoes, chicken breast, shredded ham hock or hunks of cucumber make an excellent quick ploughman's lunch with low-carb bread (see pages 101 and 124), or go Italian and take olives, cubes of Parmesan and salumi.

5 I love to pack up salads in jars, making sure the dressing is at the bottom and the most absorbent items are at the top, such as salad leaves.

6 Nuts, such as pecans, almonds, hazelnuts, brazils and macadamias, make good snacks.

7 Greek yogurt and low-carb berries.

8 Cooked oily fish, such as salmon, mackerel and sardines, are readily available and easy to eat.

9 Cooked chicken breast is easy to buy, is full of protein and will fill you up; better to have one of these than a couple of biscuits that will set sugar cravings off.

10 Run your knife around an avocado and cut to the stone, but don't pull it apart. Pack into a bag with a teaspoon and a small bottle of dressing, and you are ready to go.

11 Do hunt for well-designed lunchboxes; practical bento boxes, clip-top jars, tiffin boxes, mini jam jars and miniature bottles for dressings.

Be prepared! This is our motto so that temptation doesn't get the better of us when we are hungry and away from home.

Sohini's Spicy Sauerkraut

I was introduced to this Indian-inspired sauerkraut by our friend Sohini Basu from Calcutta. It's great to take to work with Bella's Bhajis (page 131) or make it into coleslaw with the One-Minute Mayonnaise on page 78.

Homemade sauerkraut is completely different to the vinegar-soaked shop-bought kinds. Salt in the fermenting process draws out water from the food to make a brine; a process called lacto-fermentation. Harmful bacteria cannot survive in it, but beneficial bacteria do, which is why it is so good for our guts. Gently warmed it lends a spicy, peppery zing to stir-fries or fried eggs but for maximum health benefits, do not heat sauerkraut to higher than 70°C (158°F) or you will kill the bacteria. Avoid using metal containers or utensils as the acids produced by the fermentation process could react with them. Cover your containers with vinegar-proofed lids as ordinary lids will corrode.

Wash a large, wide-mouthed jar or two in the dishwasher or with very hot soapy water, rinse them thoroughly, then allow them to cool and dry upside down on a clean rack.

Shred the cabbage, carrot and onion in a food processor or by hand. Put the vegetables, garlic and salt in a large bowl and squeeze them together with your hands until they weep plenty of water. This will be your brine.

Mix in the spices and pack the mixture into the prepared jar/s and pour in the juices from the bowl. Push the sauerkraut down under the surface with another smaller jar or a potato masher to expel most of the air inside. Add a weight on top so that the vegetables are completely submerged. If they aren't fully covered, top up the jar with some fresh brine, making sure you leave 3cm (1¼in) headspace to allow the sauerkraut to expand as it ferments. (To make more brine, dissolve 4 tablespoons of salt in 1 litre/2¾ pints filtered boiling water. Cool to room temperature and use as required).

Close the lid and set aside at room temperature for at least 3 days and up to a week depending on the warmth of your house. Check on your sauerkraut daily: skim off any thin white scum that forms on the surface and push down the vegetables, so they remain below the line of the brine. If mould appears discard the batch. Be aware that gases can build up during the fermentation process and these need to be released from time to time. Lacto-fermented foods should have a clean, slightly sour smell. Discard any that are cloudy or smell "off" and unpleasant. Trust your nose.

The sauerkraut will bubble as fermentation gets underway. Move it to the fridge after 3 days to enjoy it young and crisp or leave it to mature for longer to become more sour in flavour and softer. Store in the fridge or a cool, dark place (below 16°C/60°F is ideal).

MAKES 1.25KG (3LB)

1 white cabbage, approx. 1kg (2lb 4oz), damaged leaves and hard core discarded
1 medium carrot, approx. 75g (2¾oz)
1 medium brown onion
4 garlic cloves, finely sliced
2 tablespoons (approx. 20g/¾oz) fine salt
1 teaspoon dried oregano
1 teaspoon ground cumin
1½ teaspoons mustard seeds
½ teaspoon fennel seeds, ground

Per serving 8.4g carbs, 4.5g fibre, 1.6g protein, 0.5g fat, 51kcal

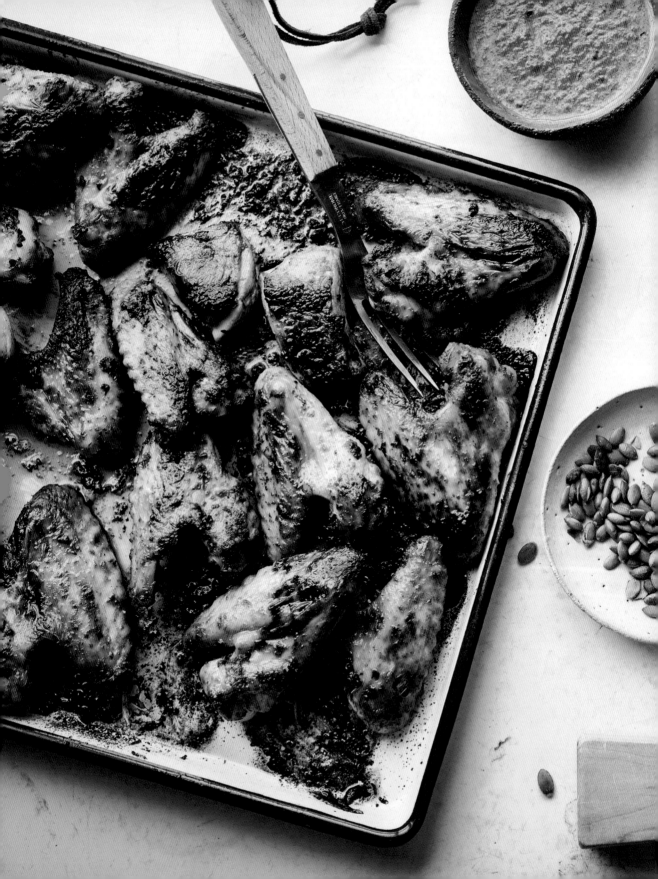

Fakeaways

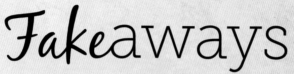

Why make your own curry, spicy chicken, burgers and chips when you can simply order in, or drive by and pick up your favourite meals? The odd treat of a takeaway is fine, but it has become all too easy for us not to cook at all and to eat highly calorific, sugar- and carb-ridden foods too frequently. The quality of takeaway food can be poor in terms of meat or fish welfare, the oils used can become toxic and the packaging extreme and unnecessary, not to mention the cost of a meal compared to the price of cooking it at home.

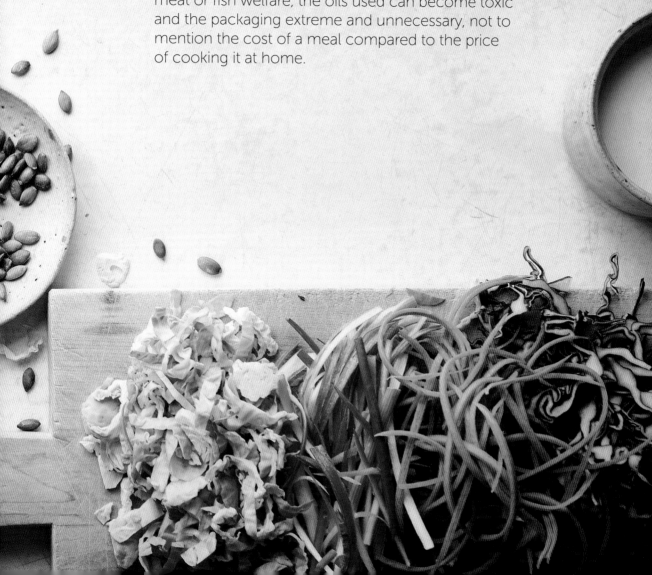

Pizza al Taglio

This is a light, airy dough and it is easier and quicker to make than traditional wheat dough; there is no rising time and the base contains a fraction of the carbs of a traditional pizza. Topping ideas are endless for Pizza al Taglio, meaning "by the slice", but I have given a few suggestions below. Don't be tempted to buy ready-grated mozzarella – some brands contain potato starch, making it higher in carbs, and it takes longer to melt.

Golden flaxseed (aka linseed) can be ground to a sandy texture in any food processor. Brown flaxseed will work fine but the colour of the base will be darker. It can become rancid in time, so it is better kept in the fridge or freezer.

Preheat the oven to 200°C/180°C fan/400°F/gas mark 6. Line a 35 x 25cm (14 x 10in) baking tray with baking parchment and lightly brush with oil.

To make the pizza base, mix the dry ingredients together in a large mixing bowl with a metal spoon. Stir in the eggs, mozzarella brine or water. When you have a well-combined dough, relax for 10 minutes and let the dough do the same. In that time the flaxseed will absorb the water. Use your hands to gather it into a ball and remove it from the bowl.

Put the dough onto the prepared tray. Press and shape it with wet hands into a rectangle just less than 1cm (½in) deep to fill the tray. Use a knife to score the pizza into 6 or 12 even divisions. Bake for 8 minutes or just until it feels firm to the touch, but don't let it brown.

Meanwhile, blend the ingredients for the sauce together with a stick blender or potato masher in a mixing bowl until smooth.

Remove the base from the oven and increase the temperature to 220°C/200°C fan/425°F/gas mark 7. Loosen the pizza from the tray just to make sure it will lift off but leave it in place. Make sure the scored lines are visible; if not, go over them again.

Top the divisions with the tomato sauce or leave some without. Add whichever toppings you wish to the sections – we like to do half of them just with a scattering of garlic, followed by some mozzarella. The rest we prefer with salami, olives and mozzarella. Mushrooms or chilli are other options. Drizzle over the olive oil.

Bake for 8–10 minutes or until the mozzarella is bubbling and the crust becomes crisp and browned. Remove from the oven and top with the tomatoes, basil, rocket and prosciutto, if using.

SERVES 6
For the flaxseed pizza base
olive oil, to grease
75g (2¾oz) golden flaxseed, ground in a food processor to a sand-like texture
100g (3½oz) ground almonds
1 teaspoon baking powder
1 teaspoon salt
1 x 125g (4½oz) ball mozzarella, coarsely grated
3 eggs, beaten
50ml (2fl oz) mozzarella brine from the bag, or water

For the tomato sauce
½ x 400g (14oz) can of tomatoes
1 teaspoon dried oregano
½ teaspoon salt
1 tablespoon extra virgin olive oil

Topping ideas
2 garlic cloves, finely chopped
1 x 125g (4½oz) mozzarella ball, drained and torn or chopped
12 black or green olives, pitted
12 slices of salami
25g (1oz) mushrooms, sliced
1 red or green chilli, finely sliced or chilli flakes, to taste
1 tablespoon extra virgin olive oil, to drizzle

To serve
cherry tomatoes, halved
a handful of basil leaves (optional)
a small handful of rocket leaves
2 slices of prosciutto (optional)

Per serving 3.5g carbs, 6.8g fibre, 21g protein, 33g fat, 409kcal

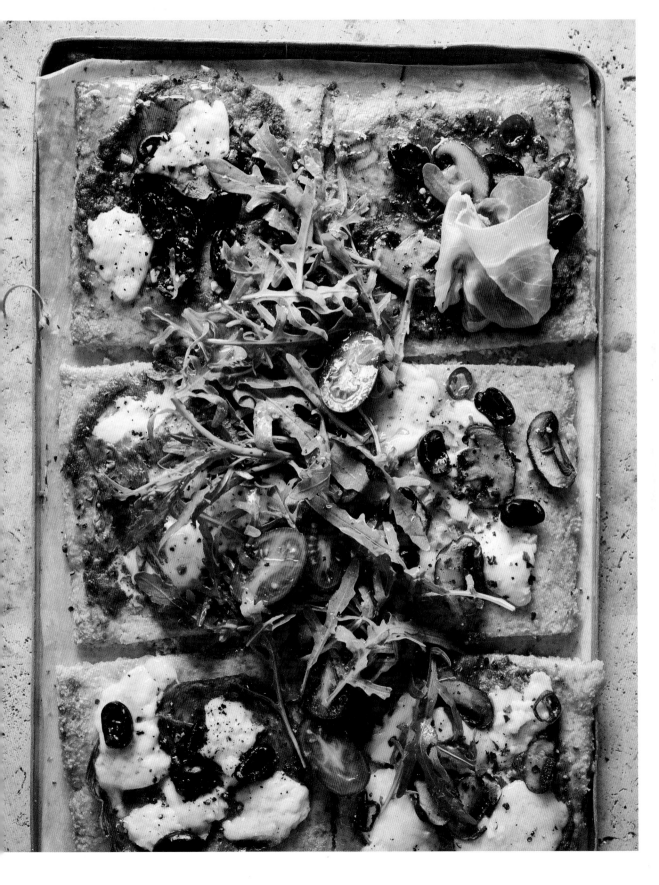

Peri-peri Chicken, Halloumi Chips & Peri-peri Dipping Sauce

By making your own Peri-peri chicken you avoid the use of refined oils and sugar. You can use any cut of chicken such as breast, wings, legs or thighs, or joint a chicken yourself and you will have something for everyone. The unused half of the pepper for the marinade can be cut into sticks and is lovely with the dip. If you have time, marinate the chicken in the sauce for 30 minutes to get the flavour into it, but it is almost as delicious cooking straight after basting. We have used a little honey to get a bit of sweetness into the sauce, but leave it out if you are very low-carb. As for the chillies, I have specified the tiny Thai bird's-eye chillies, but I have made an equally punchy sauce with 2 teaspoons of chilli flakes or large, hot red chillies. Taste the sauce as you make it and adjust the heat accordingly. Cooking will lessen the heat slightly so bump up the chillies to allow for that.

Blitz the marinade ingredients together in a food processor or chop the red pepper, garlic and chillies very finely by hand and add to the remaining ingredients. Remove one-third of the mixture and set aside for the dip.

Put the chicken pieces into a large mixing bowl and spoon over the remaining marinade. Stir through evenly, cover the bowl and put it into the fridge for 30 minutes or up to overnight (but 30 minutes is all you need).

Mix the reserved marinade with the yogurt and taste for seasoning. This will be the Peri-peri Dipping Sauce for the halloumi chips.

Preheat the oven to 220°C/200°C fan/425°F/gas mark 7. Lay the marinated chicken pieces on a roasting tray, skin side up, and cook the breast and wings for 20–30 minutes and about 45 minutes for the thighs and legs. Remove from the oven and leave to rest in a warm place for 10 minutes. Serve warm with the halloumi chips and dipping sauce alongside.

SERVES 6

1kg (2lb 4oz) chicken pieces
4 tablespoons Greek yogurt

For the marinade

½ red pepper or 3 mild red
  chillies, cored and deseeded
3 garlic cloves
4–6 red Thai bird's-eye chillies
2 teaspoons mild honey (optional)
juice of 1 lemon
2 teaspoons smoked paprika
1 teaspoon salt
4 tablespoons extra virgin olive oil

Per serving 5.9g carbs, 1.1g fibre, 31g protein, 27g fat, 390kcal

Halloumi Chips

Cut a block of halloumi cheese into chips, cubes or slices as you wish. Heat a non-stick frying pan over a medium–high heat. Add the cheese to the pan and allow to cook. Water sometimes comes out of the cheese; allow this to evaporate away. Turn the cheese when it is browned until it becomes golden all over (or at least on most sides if you made cubes). Use straight away otherwise the cheese quickly becomes firm and squeaky again.

Per 30g serving 0.5g carbs, 0g fibre, 7g protein, 7.1g fat, 93kcal

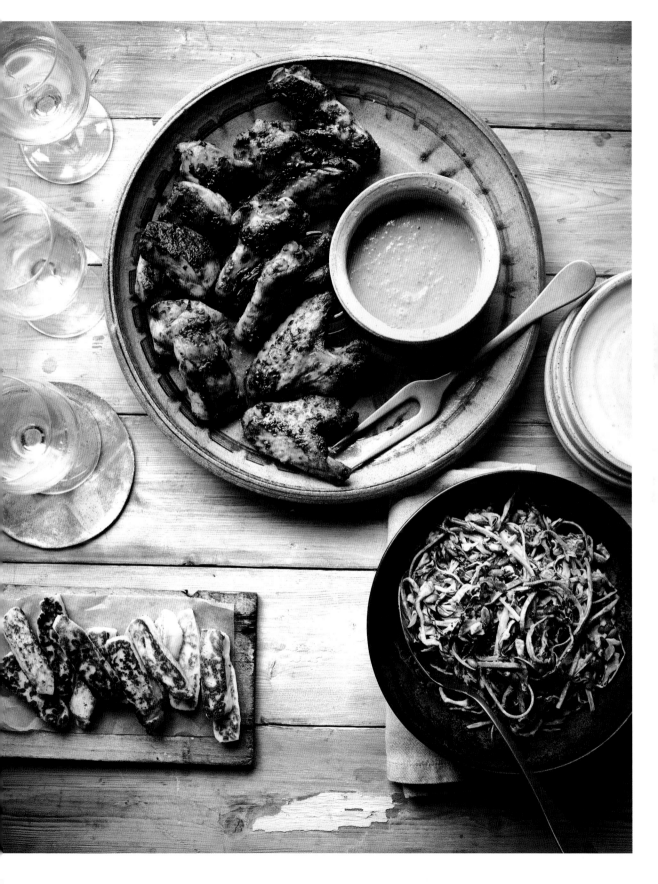

Chinese Sesame Chicken & Broccoli

This is a popular Chinese takeaway dish, but it's actually very easy to make at home. It cooks in minutes and is loved by our boys. I serve it with the Chinese Green Stir-fry (page 119) instead of white rice and everyone is happy.

Toast the sesame seeds in a dry pan until golden. Set aside on a plate and leave to cool.

Make the sauce by stirring the ingredients together in a small bowl.

Steam or boil the broccoli until just tender, then drain and set aside (to keep its colour plunge it into ice-cold water).

Make a batter by whisking together the cornflour, egg, salt, pepper, paprika and garlic in a mixing bowl. Add the chicken and stir it into the batter with a large spoon to ensure it is all well coated.

Heat the oil in a large non-stick frying pan over a medium-high heat and check that a small piece of chicken sizzles as it hits the pan. Fry the chicken pieces in the hot oil in two batches to ensure they cook through and are golden brown all over. They will take about 10 minutes. Once the first batch is done, remove the pieces from the pan with a slotted spoon and set aside on a warm plate while you cook the rest. Cut into the largest piece to check it is cooked through and not pink inside.

Once the second batch is cooked through, return the first batch of chicken and the drained broccoli to the pan and stir to combine. Pour in the sauce and heat through. When the sauce and broccoli are hot, serve in warm bowls scattered with the toasted sesame seeds.

SERVES 4

2 tablespoons sesame seeds
300g (10½oz) broccoli, cut into bite-size florets
1 tablespoon cornflour
1 egg
1 teaspoon salt
½ teaspoon freshly ground black pepper
2 teaspoons hot paprika
2 garlic cloves, grated
600g (1lb 7oz) boneless, skinless chicken breast, cut into 4cm (1½in) dice
4 tablespoons extra virgin olive oil, chicken fat or groundnut oil

For the sauce

4 tablespoons tamari or soy sauce
2 tablespoon toasted sesame oil
2 teaspoons honey
2 tablespoons Chinese rice vinegar
1 heaped tablespoon grated ginger

Per serving 10g carbs, 3.2g fibre, 43g protein, 25g fat, 441kcal

Southern-baked Chicken

For some years, Giancarlo's guilty pleasure was to eat crispy chicken late at night on his way home after work. After being told he was gluten-intolerant and had type 2 diabetes, this was no longer an option. Now, after much experimentation, our son Flavio came up with this recipe so that Giancarlo can reintroduce one of his favourite foods into his life. We love the spicy coating and serve these with wedges of lemon, coleslaw and a crisp green salad.

Preheat the oven to 200°C/180°C fan/400°F/gas mark 6. You will need a rack and a baking tray.

Mix all the ingredients for the coating in a large mixing bowl. Whisk the eggs in another large mixing bowl. Arrange in order: the chicken, egg, coating and lastly the oven rack over the tray.

Flavio calls it his "wet hand, dry hand" method, where you use one hand for the wet ingredients and one for the dry to prevent you coating your hands at the same time. Place a few pieces of chicken into the bowl with the egg, and, using one hand, toss them around until completely coated, then with the same hand, drop them into the coating without touching the mixture. Then with the other hand, mix them in the coating and place the chicken onto the oven rack. Repeat the process until all the chicken is coated. Now wash your hands.

Using a teaspoon, drizzle the oil evenly over the chicken, then place the rack one position higher than the tray so that the chicken has space to breathe and at the same time the tray will catch the juices. Bake for 25 minutes until the chicken is cooked through and the juices are no longer pink when pierced with a skewer. Let the chicken rest for 10 minutes in a warm place before serving.

MAKES 8 THIGHS

2 eggs, beaten
8 medium boneless, skinless chicken thighs (weighing about 100–130g/3½–4½oz each)
2 tablespoons olive oil, to drizzle
salt and freshly ground black pepper

For the coating

300g (10½oz) ground almonds
2 tablespoons ground ginger
1 tablespoon salt
2 tablespoons paprika
2 teaspoons freshly ground black pepper
2 tablespoons dried oregano
2 tablespoons mustard powder
2 tablespoons thyme leaves, finely chopped

Per thigh 4.3g carbs, 6.5g fibre, 36g protein, 36g fat, 496kcal

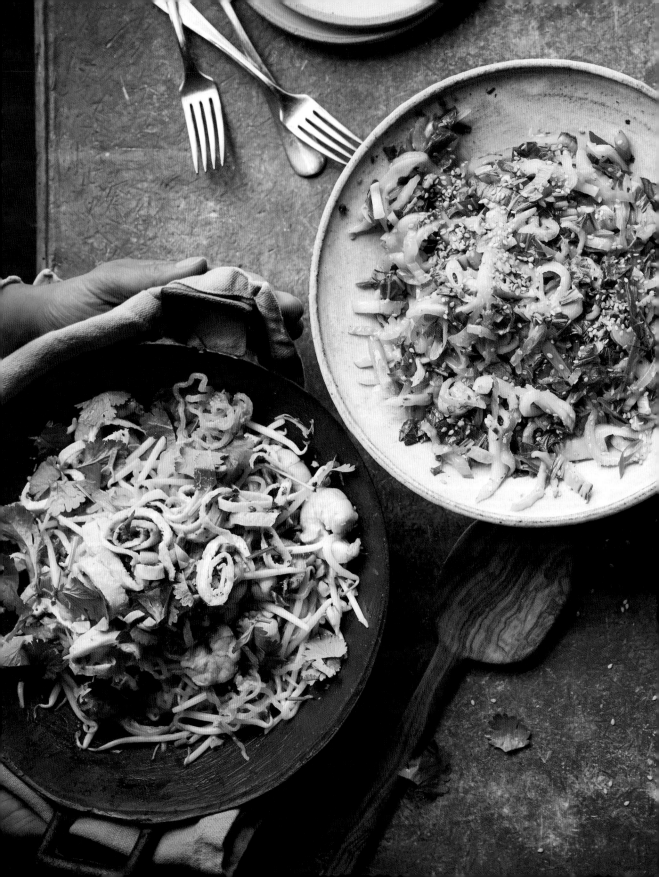

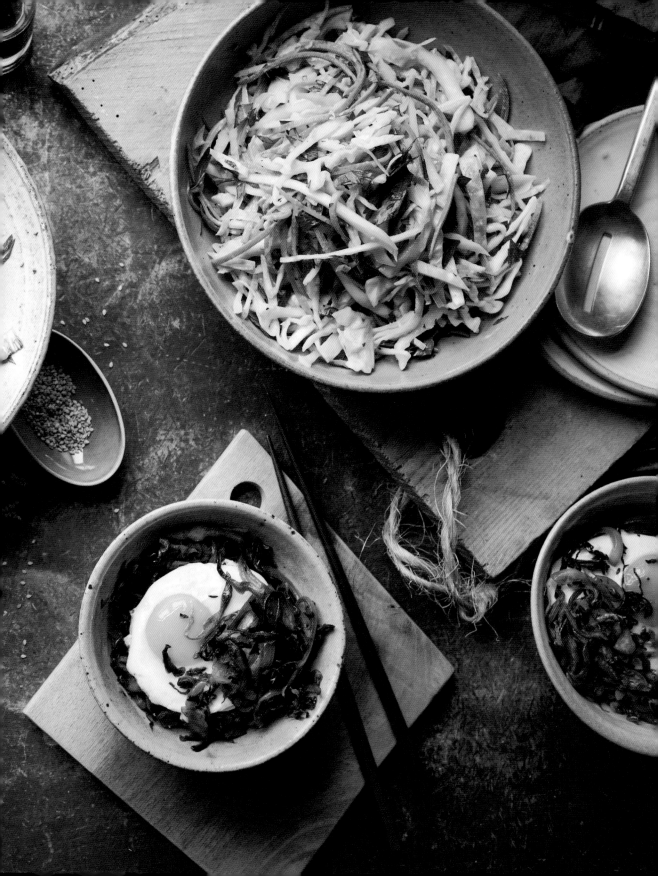

4 ways with... CABBAGE

If you look at the photo on the previous pages you will see the variety of colours of cabbages available. They have all become our friends in our low-carb lifestyle, as we use them instead of pasta, rice and potatoes. They have a fraction of the carbs and also provide plenty of fibre, vitamins and minerals.

Anna's Greek Cabbage Salad

This crunchy, light salad that our friend Anna Hudson shared with me is a traditional winter dish in Greece. Find the best kitchen gadget you can to shred the cabbage; I have a vegetable peeler or an old cheese slicer that does the trick. For large amounts it is worth using a food processor. The salad is lovely as it is or with a kick of chilli or a tablespoon of tahini.

Mix the ingredients together in a mixing bowl and season to taste. The salad will keep in the fridge for a few hours; bring to room temperature before serving.

SERVES 2

100g (3½oz) hispi, white or Chinese cabbage, very finely shredded
1 small carrot, coarsely grated
1 small garlic clove, grated
1 tablespoon lemon juice
2 tablespoons extra virgin olive oil
1 tablespoon chopped parsley
½–1 mild green chilli, finely sliced
1 tablespoon tahini (optional)
salt and freshly ground black pepper

Per serving 5.2g carbs, 4.1g fibre, 3.2g protein, 18g fat, 207kcal

Giancarlo's Red Cabbage & Apple Fry-up

Giancarlo often doesn't have time to eat when he is at work, so he loves dishes he can whip up quickly and eat in front of the footie when he gets to relax. This is one of his latest ideas – simple and quick to make, and he loves it with bacon added to the cabbage and two fried eggs.

Heat the oil in a frying pan over a medium heat and fry the onion and bacon, if using. Cook for about 7 minutes or until the onion is soft and lightly caramelized. Add the cabbage, apple, seeds and seasoning, reduce the heat to low and stir again. Put a lid on and cook for about 10 minutes or until the onion is lightly browned and the cabbage soft and tender. Taste and adjust the seasoning as necessary. Serve straight away or leave to cool and reheat when it is needed.

If you are having eggs, simply move the cabbage to one side of the pan and crack in the eggs. Fry until they are done to your liking and serve straight away.

SERVES 2

2 tablespoons extra virgin olive oil
1 small onion, finely sliced from root to tip
2 rashers of smoked streaky bacon, finely chopped (optional)
200g (7oz) red cabbage, finely shredded
1 small apple, cored and coarsely grated
½ teaspoon caraway seeds
salt and freshly ground black pepper
2 eggs (optional)

Per serving 15g carbs, 5.8g fibre, 15g protein, 24g fat, 344kcal

Pad Thai, Caldesi-style

We have replaced the traditional rice noodles with konjac noodles (see page 82). Try to find cold-pressed groundnut oil, which doesn't contain solvents and chemicals.

Have all your ingredients ready for the wok. Mix the peanut butter and honey in a bowl, then stir in the remaining sauce ingredients.

Toast the peanuts in a dry wok or large pan for 5 minutes or until golden brown. Roughly crush using a pestle and mortar, or chop by hand; set aside.

In another small bowl, beat the egg and season. Add 1 tablespoon of the oil to the wok or a large frying pan over a high heat and swirl it around to cover the base. Add the egg and swirl the pan again to spread it around creating a thin omelette. Scatter over 1 tablespoon of the coriander leaves. Flip the omelette to briefly cook the other side. Transfer to a plate and leave to cool.

Heat the remaining oil and let it get hot. Add the spring onions and chilli, then shake the wok and stir continuously for 2 minutes. Add the prawns and keep frying until they turn pink. Stir in the cabbage and stir-fry for 1 minute. Add the beansprouts and noodles, using tongs to combine everything. Now move the ingredients to the outside of the wok, leaving a circle in the centre. Pour in the sauce and bring to the boil. Bubble fast for 1 minute, then combine it with the ingredients from the outside.

Roll up the omelette and cut into ribbons. Stir it into the noodles. Serve in warm bowls with the remaining coriander and the crushed peanuts.

SERVES 2

25g (1oz) unroasted peanuts
1 egg
3 tablespoons groundnut oil
a small handful of coriander leaves, stems finely chopped
3 spring onions, finely sliced
1 red Thai chilli, finely chopped
225g (8oz) raw king prawns
150g (5½oz) cabbage, very finely shredded
200g (7oz) beansprouts, fresh or canned (drained weight)
250g (9oz) konjac noodles, drained

For the sauce

1 tablespoon peanut butter
2 teaspoons honey
juice of ½ lime
2 tablespoons tamari or soy sauce
2 garlic cloves, grated
15g (1oz) ginger, grated
1 teaspoon fish sauce
1 teaspoon toasted sesame oil

Per serving 22g carbs, 7.1g fibre, 38g protein, 30g fat, 523kcal

Chinese Green Stir-fry

Use vegetables such as cabbage, mangetout, green pepper, green beans, pak choi or broccoli for this recipe. This makes the ideal side dish to the Chinese Spare Ribs on page 135 or the Chinese Sesame Chicken & Broccoli on page 114.

Dry-fry the sesame seeds in a wok until golden. Tip onto a plate to cool.

Heat the oil in a large wok or non-stick frying pan over a high heat. Add the chilli, garlic and ginger and fry for a minute. Then add the onions and fry for 2 minutes. Lastly, add the vegetables and stir constantly, keeping the pan over a high heat for 4–5 minutes until the vegetables become tender but still have some bite. Stir in the Chinese rice wine and sesame oil. Season to taste and serve scattered with the toasted sesame seeds.

SERVES 2

1 tablespoon sesame seeds
2 tablespoons groundnut oil
⅛–¼ hot green chilli, sliced
2 fat garlic cloves, finely grated
15g (1oz) ginger, finely grated
5 spring onions, finely sliced
300g (10½oz) green vegetables, finely sliced
1 tablespoon Chinese rice wine
1 teaspoon toasted sesame oil
salt and freshly ground black pepper

Per serving 14g carbs, 7.4g fibre, 6g protein, 23g fat, 312kcal

Carnitas

Robbie and Rose Ford are keen visitors to their local taco joints in Los Angeles where they pick up tips, tricks and the latest trends. They love to cook carnitas as it is a great recipe to make in a big batch, then reheat to serve to friends. The carnitas keep for up to 5 days in the fridge. The tortillas, sauce and salsa can also be made in advance and kept in covered containers for up to 2 days in the fridge.

Preheat the oven to 170°C/150°C fan/340°F/gas mark 3½.

Soak the chillies in the hot water for about 20 minutes or until soft. Cut away and discard the skin on the pork shoulder, but leave any fat intact. Cut into 5cm (2in) pieces.

Use a pestle and mortar to lightly crush the cloves, allspice and cumin, or put the spices on a chopping board and crush using a bottle or rolling pin.

Remove the chillies from the water and finely chop them. Keep the water.

Put all the ingredients into a large casserole dish, including the reserved chilli water, and stir to combine. Cover with a lid or foil and put into the oven for 3 hours. Meanwhile, make Rose's sauce and Robbie's salsa.

Remove the casserole from the oven and use two forks to lift the meat onto a chopping board. Reserve the sauce. Pull and tear the meat with the forks into rough shreds.

Sieve the leftover tomato sauce from the meat into a jug and pour about half of it into a large frying pan over a high heat. Add the meat, a little at a time, and cook it until it is crisp and sticky. Transfer to a serving dish to keep warm. Add more sauce to the pan as necessary and reheat all the meat or as much as you need at that time.

SERVES 10

1 dried ancho chilli
1 dried smoked chipotle chilli
250ml (9fl oz) hot water
1.8kg (4lb) pork shoulder
4 cloves
10 allspice berries
1 teaspoon cumin seeds
3 fat garlic cloves, lightly crushed
2 oranges, 3 long strips of peel and the juice of 2
2 onions, each cut into 6 wedges
2 teaspoons dried oregano
2 bay leaves
1 x 12cm (4½in) cinnamon stick, snapped in half
2 teaspoons salt
plenty of freshly ground black pepper
400g (14oz) can of Italian plum tomatoes, roughly crushed

To serve

Rose's Green & Lovely Sauce (see below)
Robbie's Hot Salsa Roja (page 122)
Soft Tortillas (page 122)
a handful of shredded red cabbage
2 limes, cut into wedges
a handful of coriander
queso fresco or feta cheese, shaved

Per serving 6.1g carbs, 1.3g fibre, 42g protein, 29g fat, 460kcal

Rose's Green & Lovely Sauce

SERVES 10
2 medium avocados, roughly chopped
100g (3½oz) soured cream
1–2 jalapeño or Thai bird's-eye chillies
juice of 2 limes
25g (1oz) coriander leaves and stalks
salt and freshly ground black pepper

Whizz all the ingredients together in a food processor until smooth.

Season to taste.

Per serving 1g carbs, 0.8g protein, 8g fat, 1g fibre, 83kcal

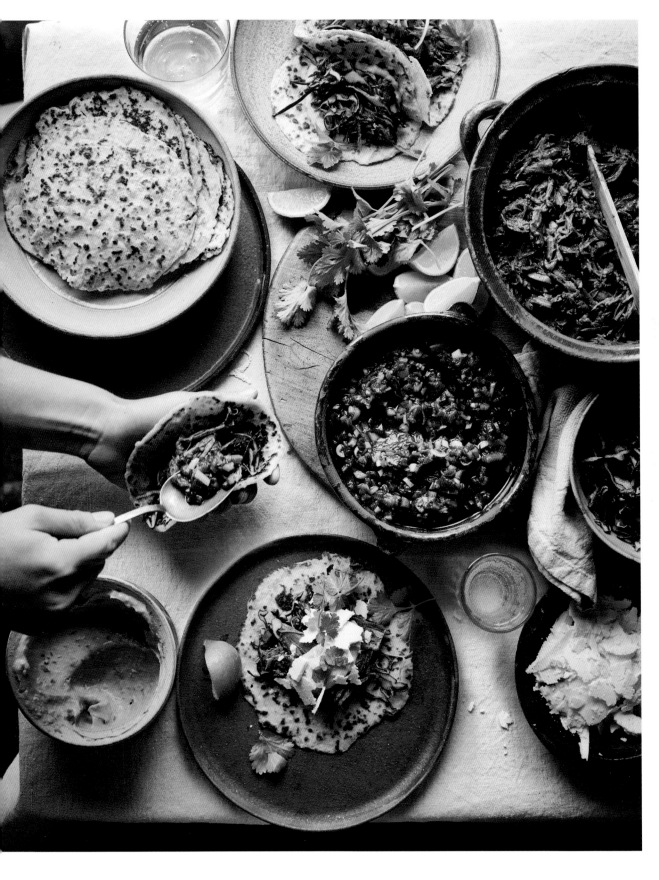

Soft Tortillas

This is our way of making soft tortillas, which are normally made of corn and hefty on the carbs. Our version comes in at 4.3g carbs per tortilla compared to your average corn version at up to 30g.

Blitz all the ingredients, except the fat, together in a blender until you have a smooth batter. You can also do this by hand with a whisk in a bowl. Leave the batter to stand for 10 minutes.

Warm a little fat in a crêpe or non-stick frying pan about 20cm (8in) in diameter over a fairly high heat. Pour in 40ml (about 3 tablespoons) of the mixture. Swirl and spread the batter out a little with a spatula to form an even round pancake. When cooked to golden brown and set on one side, usually about 3 minutes, flip the wrap over using a spatula and cook the other side for a further minute or two. Tip onto a plate when both sides are cooked and keep warm while you continue to make the rest.

MAKES 16

2 eggs
80g (2¾oz) chickpea (gram) flour
60g (2¼oz) flaxseed, ground
60g (2¼oz) ground almonds
500ml (18fl oz) whole milk
½ teaspoon salt
ghee, chicken fat or groundnut oil, to fry

Per tortilla 4.3g carbs, 2.2g fibre, 4.9g protein, 5.9g fat, 94kcal

Robbie's Hot Salsa Roja

This spicy tomato and chilli salsa was shown to us by Robbie; it is easy to throw together and pairs perfectly with his wife Rose's sauce (page 120). Whatever chilli you use, make sure you taste it first so that it gives the right spicy kick to the tacos or the Nachos on page 138.

SERVES 8–10

6 spring onions or 1 small onion, roughly chopped
1–2 jalapeños or other hot green chillies, stems removed and roughly chopped
250g (9oz) small tomatoes, top core removed or 400g (14oz) can of Italian plum tomatoes, drained
2 garlic cloves, split and crushed
2 tablespoons extra virgin olive oil
½ teaspoon smoked chipotle or normal chilli powder (optional)
1 tablespoon cider or red wine vinegar or 2 tablespoons lime juice
salt and freshly ground black pepper

Finely chop the onions, chilli, tomatoes and garlic by hand or whizz together in a food processor. Stir in the remaining ingredients and season to taste.

Per serving 1.8g carbs, 0.7g fibre, 0.5g protein, 2.6g fat, 36kcal

The Burger

It's easy to buy ready-minced beef off the shelf, but a quick visit to a butcher's counter will introduce you to different cuts that change the flavour, the fat content and value. We like to use skirt, chuck or stewing beef. Normally, these cuts need time to break down, but by mincing them they are perfect for burgers. Our chef, Stefano Borella, adds spicy, savoury Worcestershire sauce to his burgers, which we love. Make up the burgers just before cooking or the salt can make the burgers tough.

Mix the beef mince with the salt and Worcestershire sauce, if using. Divide the mixture into 4 even-sized balls and use wetted hands to form them into patties roughly 12cm (4½in) in diameter and 1cm (½in) deep. They should be at room temperature to ensure even cooking.

Heat the fat in a non-stick frying pan and, when hot enough to make a small piece of the meat sizzle, cook the burgers for 1 minute, then turn and cook for 2–3 minutes or until cooked through. (If cheese is one of your serving options, it is best to put this on top of the burgers as soon as you turn them, then put a lid on the pan to keep enough heat inside to melt it.) They are now ready to assemble (see page 124).

MAKES 4 BURGERS

500g (1lb 2oz) beef mince (15%-fat chuck, skirt or stewing beef), coarsely minced
1 teaspoon salt
1 tablespoon Worcestershire sauce (optional)
1 tablespoon lard, butter, ghee or extra virgin olive oil, to fry

Extras

Sesame Buns (see overleaf)
Tomato Relish (see below)
100g (3½oz) mature Cheddar, finely sliced (optional)
fried onions
gherkins, sliced
1 large slicing tomato, thinly sliced
lettuce leaves

Per burger 1.3g carbs, 0g fibre, 27g protein, 8.7g fat, 193kcal

The Tomato Relish

This easy, sugar-free relish can be left rough or puréed until smooth to resemble ketchup. It will keep in a glass jar or bottle in your fridge for up to a week.

SERVES 12/mMakes approx. 200ml (7fl oz)

1 small red onion, finely chopped
2 tablespoons extra virgin olive oil
2 garlic cloves, finely chopped
½ x 400g (14oz) can of chopped tomatoes
200g (7oz) fresh tomatoes, finely diced
¼–½ teaspoon chilli powder
2 teaspoons balsamic or red wine vinegar
2 teaspoons soy sauce or a good pinch of salt

Soften the onion in the oil in a small pan over a low heat until it is tender but not browned. Add the garlic and continue to cook for 2 minutes, then add the rest of the ingredients and stir through. Bring to the boil, then reduce the heat to low and simmer for 20 minutes or until the volume has halved. Taste and adjust the seasoning. Allow to cool before storing.

Per serving 1.9g carbs, 0.5g fibre, 0.5g protein, 2.2g fat, 31kcal

The Sesame Bun

This bread lasts for 3 days in the bread bin and freezes well. Psyllium husk is full of fibre and binds the dough; it is available from health-food shops and online. However, it should be a fine powder and will measure differently if it is still coarse; pulse it in a food processor for a couple of minutes to break it down. Some types of psyllium husk give the bread a dark purple colour; it you'd prefer pale brown bread, buy blond psyllium husk instead. Further flavourings, such as 2 teaspoons of finely chopped rosemary and stoned black olives, make a wonderful addition to the bread and are in the photo of the Antipasti Salad on page 32.

Preheat the oven to 220°C/200°C fan/425°F/gas mark 7. Grease a baking tray with a little olive oil.

Mix all the dry ingredients together in a mixing bowl. Add the eggs and stir through briefly with a metal spoon. Add the boiling water and stir through quickly until you have a well-combined mixture. (You can also do this in a stand mixer or food processor.) Remove the dough from the bowl and drizzle a little oil on your hands.

Divide the dough into 4 x 100g (3½oz) balls and, using wetted hands, roll and then flatten into discs about 10cm (4in) across. Alternatively, create 8 x 50g (1¾oz) balls and flatten them to about 7cm (2¾in) diameter. Place them on the prepared tray and top each one with a few sesame seeds. Bake for 25–30 minutes or until the rolls feel light to the touch and come off the tray easily. Allow to cool to room temperature before cutting or eating. The buns will keep in the fridge in a sealed container for up to 5 days. They can be toasted or heated in the microwave or oven.

MAKES 4 LARGE OR 8 SMALLER BUNS

olive oil, to grease the tray and shape the dough
150g (5½oz) ground almonds
5 tablespoons (25g/1oz) ground psyllium husk powder
2 teaspoons baking powder
½ teaspoon fine sea salt
3 eggs
250ml (9fl oz) boiling water
1 tablespoon sesame seeds

Per large (10cm/4in) bun
3.5g carbs, 25g fibre, 17g protein, 27g fat, 369kcal

Per small (7cm/2¾in) bun
1.7g carbs, 12g fibre, 8.3g protein, 13g fat, 184kcal

To assemble
Cut the sesame buns in half and spread the relish onto the base. Put the burger on top with melted cheese, if using, some fried onions, sliced gherkins, a slice of tomato and lettuce. Add the tops of the buns and serve straight away.

To make your own burger relish

Mix together 100ml (3½fl oz) Tomato Relish (page 123), 100ml (3½fl oz) One-minute Mayonnaise (page 98) or Hellmann's mayonnaise, 50ml (2fl oz) wholegrain or American yellow mustard and 50g (1¾oz) finely chopped gherkins. Adjust the flavours with extra mustard or gherkins as you like and serve straight away. A jar of your own burger relish will last up to a week in the fridge. This makes enough for 10 burgers.

Per serving 0.9g carbs, 0.5g fibre, 0.7g protein, 8.9g fat, 88kcal

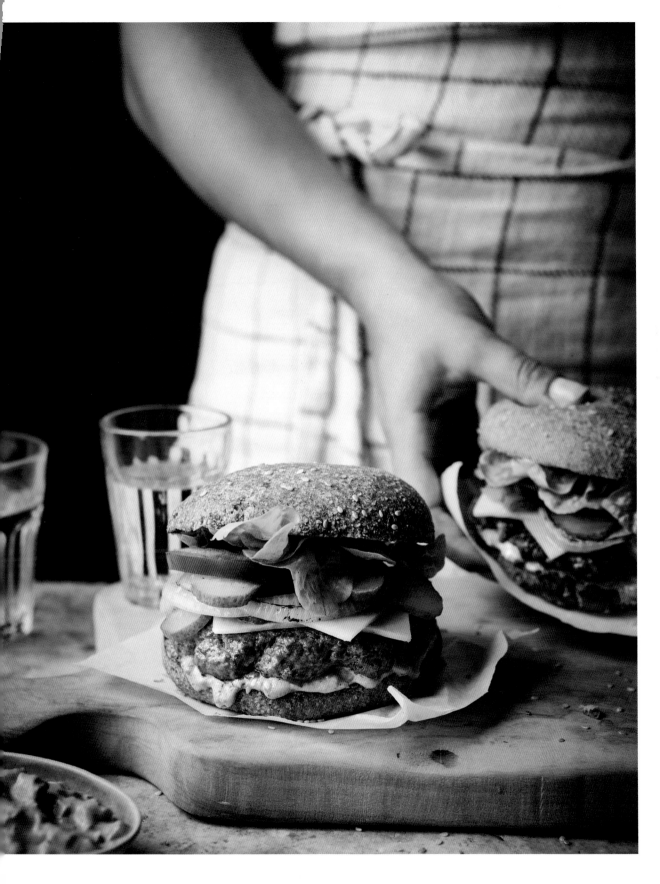

Thai Red Beef Curry

Always a popular choice at the local Thai takeaway, this curry balances the sweetness from the coconut with the heat of the chilli. This is often cooked quickly, but we love slow-cooked meat. It means you can use a less expensive cut, which often has more flavour and you can get on with something else while the flavours slowly combine in the oven. We have added swede as, although it is a root vegetable, it isn't too high in carbs; it bumps up the volume so that you can eat this on its own in bowls rather than needing the traditional white rice alongside, although you could have it with Cauli-Rice (page 66), konjac noodles (see page 82), or the Chinese Green Stir-fry (page 119).

We have worked with several Thai chefs over the years and picked up tips on creating the best flavour in curry sauces such as this. We have used dried red chillies, but you could use fresh bird's-eye, standard red chilli or chilli flakes or powder; the point is to get the heat that will, in the end, be toned down by the coconut. It is impossible to be prescriptive about how many chillies to use, as I have no idea what shape, size and heat yours possess, so I can give a rough guide but you must taste and adjust to your liking and the heat in your chillies. If you want to speed things up, use a good shop-bought Thai red curry paste.

Preheat the oven to 170°C/150°C fan/340°F/gas mark 3½.

Traditionally, ingredients for a curry paste are pounded in a pestle and mortar and that is the way I was shown. However, I must admit I now whizz all the ingredients together in a small food processor with 2–3 tablespoons of water to help it blend. Alternatively, you can finely chop the ingredients together by hand and then mix together without the water.

Select a large ovenproof casserole dish with a lid in which to heat the oil over a high heat and fry the garlic, ginger and lemongrass for 2 minutes. Add the curry paste and stir through, allowing it to bubble and splutter for 2 minutes. Add the salt and coconut milk and stir through. Bring to the boil and stir in the meat, swede and stock. Bring to the boil again, put on the lid and transfer to the oven for 2½ hours or until the beef and swede are soft. Taste the sauce and adjust the seasoning as necessary. Serve scattered with the coriander leaves and the lime wedges alongside.

SERVES 6

For the Thai red curry paste
8 dried chillies, soaked in hot water for 10 minutes, then drained or fresh, roughly chopped
½ teaspoon ground cumin
½ teaspoon ground coriander
1 shallot, roughly chopped
8 medium garlic cloves
½ teaspoon salt
25g (1oz) ginger, peeled
1 lemongrass stalk, roughly chopped
5 kaffir lime leaves
2 teaspoons fish sauce

For the curry
3 tablespoons cold-pressed groundnut oil or coconut oil
2 fat garlic cloves, finely chopped
15g (½oz) ginger, peeled and finely chopped
1 lemongrass stalk, finely sliced
½ teaspoon salt
400ml (14fl oz) can coconut milk
1kg (2lb 4oz) flank, skirt or stewing steak, cut into approx. 1 x 5cm (½–2in) pieces
350g (12oz) swede, peeled and cut into 1 x 5cm (½–2in) pieces
200ml (7fl oz) beef stock or hot water

To serve
a small handful of coriander leaves
lime wedges

Per serving 7.2g carbs, 1.6g fibre, 41g protein, 35g fat, 505kcal

Lamb Rogan Josh

This is one of the most popular takeaway dishes from Indian restaurants and yet it isn't difficult to make at home. Don't be put off by the list of ingredients. After a simple spooning of spices into the mix, you are ready to cook. Then you just need to give the ingredients time and they will be transformed into a wonderful rich curry. We have given the option of using mutton or lamb, the former being my preference, as it is inexpensive, underused and full of flavour. Serve with the Turmeric Cauli-Rice (page 66). The curry can be cooked in the oven if you prefer: give it the same length of time and cook it at 170°C/150°C fan/340°F/gas mark 3½.

Toast the cumin, coriander, fennel, cloves, if using, and fenugreek briefly in a dry frying pan until they release their aroma. Use a pestle and mortar to grind briefly and break them up.

Heat half the ghee in a large, heavy-based pan over a high heat. When hot, brown the lamb in two batches until brown all over. Don't crowd the pan and expect this to take about 20 minutes. Remove the meat and set aside on a plate.

Reduce the heat and add the remaining ghee to the pan. When hot, add the garlic, ginger and onions, stir through and cook over a gentle heat for about 10 minutes.

Add the meat and all the spices to the onions with the salt. Stir regularly and cook for 5 minutes. Add the tomato purée and 500ml (18fl oz) of the stock and bring to the boil.

Reduce the heat so that the curry simmers gently for 1½ hours for lamb and 2½ hours for mutton. Add a little more stock as necessary so that it doesn't dry out. Now stir in the yogurt and cream and taste for seasoning. Serve straight away or allow to cool before storing. The curry will keep in the fridge for 4 days.

SERVES 6

2 teaspoons cumin seeds
2 teaspoons coriander seeds
1 teaspoon fennel seeds
½ teaspoon cloves (optional)
½ teaspoon fenugreek seeds
4 tablespoons ghee or olive oil
1kg (2lb 4oz) boneless stewing lamb or mutton, cut into pieces
4 garlic cloves, grated
25g (1oz) ginger, grated
2 onions, finely chopped
8 cardamom pods, split open
½ teaspoon ground turmeric
2 teaspoons chilli powder
½ teaspoon asafoetida (optional)
1 cinnamon stick, snapped in half
2 teaspoons salt
3 tablespoons tomato purée
500–750ml (18fl oz–1¼ pints) hot chicken, beef or vegetable stock or water
75g (2¾oz) whole Greek yogurt
75ml (2¾fl oz) double cream
salt and freshly ground black pepper

Per serving 8.9g carbs, 2.5g fibre, 47g protein, 35g fat, 547kcal

Chicken Tikka Masala

This chicken recipe works in two ways: it is lovely as a spicy, dry tikka or deliciously creamy in the masala sauce. We like the chicken tikka hot or cold with salad and the chicken tikka masala with Turmeric Cauli-Rice (page 66).

Cut the chicken into even, bite-sized pieces. Put into a mixing bowl and season. Add the remaining tikka ingredients to the bowl and stir through to coat the pieces. Put in the fridge to marinate for 30 minutes. Line a baking tray with foil and brush with oil or ghee.

Meanwhile, make the sauce. Melt the butter in a saucepan over a medium-low heat. Add the onion and garlic. Cook for a few minutes, and when the onion is soft, add the spices and chilli and fry until aromatic. Add the tomatoes and cook down for 10 minutes. Blend until smooth in a food processor or with a stick blender. Stir in the cream, season to taste and cook over a low heat for 5–10 minutes.

Preheat the grill to high. Put the chicken pieces on the prepared tray and spread out evenly. Cook high under the grill for 15 minutes or until cooked through. Do keep an eye on the chicken so that the pieces don't burn, but a little light charring is good for flavour.

Remove the chicken from the grill and serve as it is or add to the saucepan. Stir through and serve hot, scattered with the coriander.

SERVES 6

For the chicken tikka
4–6 boneless, skinless chicken breasts, approx. 800g (1lb 2oz)
zest and juice of ½ lemon
2 garlic cloves
10g (¼oz) ginger, peeled and grated
1 teaspoon chilli powder or flakes
½ teaspoon ground turmeric
½ teaspoon ground cumin
½ teaspoon ground coriander
1 green chilli, finely chopped
50g (1¾oz) double cream
50g (1¾oz) Greek yogurt
salt and freshly ground black pepper
oil or melted ghee, to grease

For the masala sauce
15g (½oz) butter
1 onion, finely chopped
3 garlic cloves, grated
15g (½oz) ginger, grated
1 teaspoon coriander seeds
1 teaspoon cumin seeds
4 cardamom pods
1 teaspoon paprika
½ teaspoon fenugreek seeds
1 green chilli, split in half
400g (14oz) can of tomatoes
100ml (3½fl oz) double cream
coriander, leaves picked and stalks finely chopped, to serve

Per serving (chicken tikka)
0.8g carbs, 0g fibre, 42g protein, 11g fat, 277kcal
Per serving (chicken tikka masala)
6.1g carbs, 1.3g fibre, 43g protein, 22g fat, 409kcal

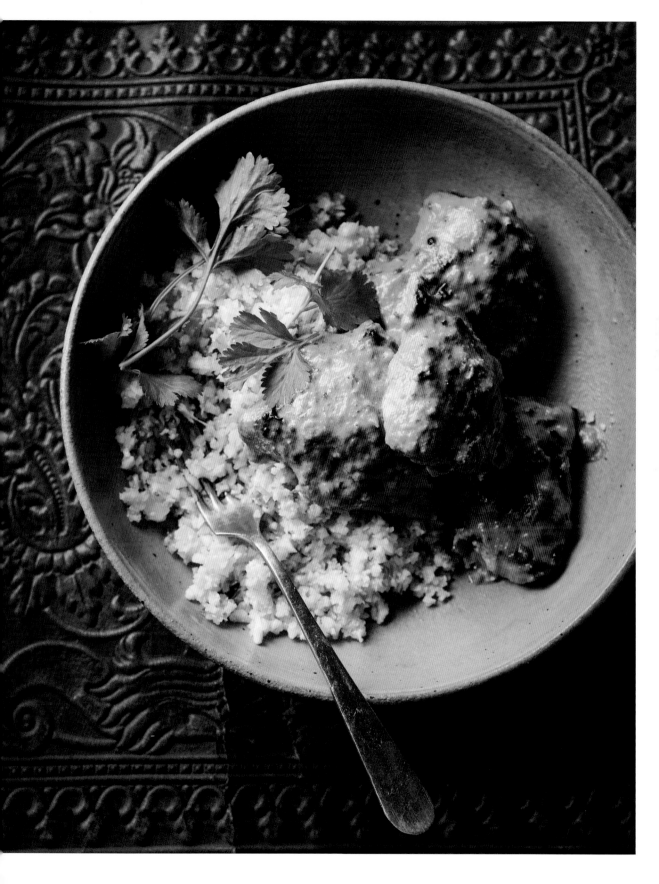

Shilpi's Cauliflower Muttar Paneer

Shilpi Prasad is from near Kolkata and, like most north Indians, she uses ghee for cooking (in the south they use coconut oil). She is vegetarian and uses peanuts, almonds or cashews to add protein, fat and texture to the "gravy" as she calls the sauce. Shilpi doesn't include chilli but you can add it to your taste. Do read through the recipe first; it seems long but it is actually quite simple. Mushrooms or spinach can be added instead of peas or add thin strips of pepper 5 minutes before the end. Shilpi told me many of the herbs and spices are optional, so if you don't have one or two, leave them out. We love this in bowls with halved boiled eggs, Bella's Bhajis (opposite) or alongside a meat curry.

Heat one-quarter of the fat in a large non-stick frying pan or wok over a high heat. Add the garlic and onions and stir to make sure they are well coated in the fat. Put a lid on top and let them cook for 5 minutes, shaking the pan every now and again. Continue cooking for about 7 minutes or until they are soft. Remove from the heat and set aside on a plate to cool.

Clean the pan with kitchen paper and heat another quarter of the fat in it over a high heat. Add the cumin seeds and chilli, if using, and after a minute add the cauliflower. Stir through and cover with a lid, turn the heat to medium and cook the cauliflower for 5 minutes.

Meanwhile, blend the garlic, onions and peanuts to a paste in a blender, adding a splash of water, if necessary, to help them blend.

Tip the cauliflower florets out onto a plate once they are lightly browned. Add another quarter of the fat to the pan and allow to foam over a low heat. When it foams, add the bay leaves and cardamom pod/s followed by the paste (don't wash the blender). Stir through, then add the ground spices and salt and stir through. Cook the paste for 5 minutes.

Meanwhile, unless using passata, purée the tomatoes to a smooth consistency. Add to the pan with the curry and chilli powders and bring to the boil. Taste and add a little more if you like. Put the lid on to avoid splashes and cook for 5 minutes.

Now add the peas, cauliflower and paneer to the pan and stir through. Put the lid on and cook for a further 10 minutes or so until the cauliflower is just tender. If the sauce looks very dry, add the water to thin it to your liking. Taste the curry for seasoning and adjust accordingly. Add the last knob of the fat and stir through to make it glossy.

Add the coriander stalks and stir through. Scatter the leaves on top and stir through, then serve straight away.

SERVES 4

30g (1oz) ghee or butter or 3 tablespoons extra virgin olive oil

3 fat garlic cloves, roughly chopped

3 medium onions, roughly sliced into half moons

1 teaspoon cumin seeds

1 hot red or green chilli, halved (optional)

400g (14oz) (½ large one) cauliflower, cut into bite-size florets

30g (1oz) roasted peanuts, with or without skin

2 bay leaves

1 black cardamom pod or 2 green ones, lightly crushed (seeds discarded)

½–1 teaspoon ground turmeric, added according to colour

1 heaped teaspoon ground coriander

½ teaspoon ground cumin

½ teaspoon ground fenugreek seeds

1½ teaspoons salt

400g (14oz) passata or can of tomatoes, or 4 fresh tomatoes, roughly chopped

1–2 teaspoons masala curry powder

½–1 teaspoon chilli powder

100g (3½oz) frozen peas

200g (7oz) paneer, diced into 2cm (¾in) cubes

100-150ml (3½–5fl oz) water

a small handful of coriander, leaves picked and stalks finely chopped (optional)

Per serving 28g carbs, 8g fibre, 23g protein, 27g fat, 464kcal

Bella's Bhajis with Coriander & Mint Raita

These really shouldn't have been Bella's bhajis, as she is our dog, but you can guess the rest. Now every time I make them, she circles around me expectantly. Instead of deep-frying, we like to oven bake the patties to give them a light, crunchy finish. We add a kick of chilli to the bhajis, but you can omit this or add any kind of chilli that you have that has a punch. I can't be prescriptive about the amount, as chillies differ so much; you have to taste them and add accordingly. The bhajis are ideal with any of the curries in the book or as canapés if you make them half the size (reduce the cooking time by 5 minutes) and top them with the dip and a coriander leaf. I have given the option of parsley rather than coriander, as we have a coriander-loather in our household; it is a genetic variant, so I can't call him fussy!

First make the raita. Mix all the ingredients together. Taste and adjust the seasoning. Transfer to a serving bowl, cover and keep chilled until you are ready to serve.

Preheat the oven to 200°C/180°C fan/400°F/gas mark 6. Prepare a baking tray by greasing it generously with 2 teaspoons of the oil.

Whisk the chickpea and coconut flours, salt, cumin seeds, curry powder and baking powder together in a mixing bowl, then gradually add the water to form a thick batter. Add the remaining ingredients, including the remaining olive oil, and stir to combine.

Now dollop 12 even-sized mounds of the mixture onto the prepared tray and flatten gently to form round patties about 7cm (2¾in) in diameter. Bake for 20 minutes, then use a metal slice to turn them gently to cook on the other side for 10–15 minutes or until set firm and golden brown on both sides. Serve warm or at room temperature with the raita, scattered with extra coriander or parsley leaves.

MAKES 12 BHAJIS

3 tablespoons extra virgin olive oil
60g (2¼oz) chickpea (gram) flour
20g (¾oz) coconut flour
¾ teaspoon salt
1 heaped teaspoon cumin seeds
1 heaped teaspoon masala curry powder
1 teaspoon baking powder
200–250ml (7–9fl oz) water
100g (3½oz) leek, halved lengthways, then cut into half moons
50g (1¾oz) baby spinach leaves, roughly chopped
20g (¾oz) coriander or parsley, leaves roughly chopped and stalks finely chopped, plus extra leaves to serve
1 hot green chilli, finely chopped, or ½ teaspoon chilli flakes

For the raita (serves 6)

200g (7oz) Greek yogurt
a handful of mint leaves, finely chopped
a handful of coriander or parsley leaves, finely chopped, plus a few extra leaves to serve
1 teaspoon ground cumin
juice of ½ lemon
salt

Per bhaji 3.2g carbs, 1.4g fibre, 1.7g protein, 3.7g fat, 56kcal
Per serving of raita 1.7g carbs, 0g fibre, 2g protein, 3.4g fat, 46kcal

Chicken Shawarma

Shawarma means "turning", a reference to the turning pile of chicken in front of the heat at any kebab shop. This method of making the dish was shown to me by our Kuwaiti friend Amal, who keeps the chicken tender by cooking it in a frying pan with a lid.

Separate the layers of red onion and put them into a small bowl with cold water to cover; set aside, soaking will take the strength of the onion away.

Heat the oil in a large frying pan and, when hot, add the onion, breaking it up with your fingers to separate the layers, followed by the garlic and chilli. Fry over a medium heat, stirring frequently, until the onion starts to soften. Stir through the chicken, the seasoning, spices and tomatoes.

Cook over a low heat, covered, for about 10 minutes, then remove the lid and continue to cook for a further 10 minutes or until the chicken is cooked through (check that the largest piece of chicken is not pink inside). Remove the lid and taste for seasoning and the heat of the chilli, adjusting as necessary. Transfer the chicken into a warm serving dish.

Meanwhile, make the sauce by whisking the ingredients together in a bowl until smooth, diluting it with enough water to achieve a pouring consistency. Pour into a jug to serve. It will keep in the fridge for a week.

Drain the red onion and serve alongside the warm chicken topped with parsley or coriander, the tahini sauce, chillies, sugar-free chilli sauce, pitta or flatbreads and Anna's Greek Cabbage Salad (page 118).

SERVES 8

1 red onion, finely sliced
3 tablespoons extra virgin olive oil
1 onion, finely sliced into half
  moons
4 garlic cloves, finely chopped
½–1 green or red chilli, finely
  chopped, or 1 teaspoon chilli
  flakes
1kg (2lb 4oz) boneless, skinless
  chicken breasts, cut into finger-
  width lengths
2 teaspoons salt
generous twists of freshly ground
  black pepper
½ teaspoon ground turmeric
1 heaped teaspoon paprika
1 teaspoon ground coriander
½ teaspoon ground cinnamon
2 teaspoons ground cumin
1–2 large tomatoes (approx.
  150g/5½oz), roughly chopped
a large handful of parsley or
  coriander, roughly chopped

For the tahini sauce

3 tablespoons extra virgin olive oil
1 garlic clove, finely chopped
3 tablespoons tahini
2 tablespoons Greek yogurt
juice of ½ lemon
good pinch of salt and freshly
  ground black pepper
2–3 tablespoons water, as needed

Per serving of shawarma
3.8g carbs, 1.1g fibre, 31g protein,
6.2g fat, 196kcal

Per serving of tahini sauce
0.7g carbs, 0.6g fibre, 2.2g protein,
10g fat, 103kcal

Per pitta 1.7g carbs, 12g fibre,
7.9g protein, 12g fat, 174kcal

Per flatbread 2.3g carbs, 12g fibre,
8.2g protein, 16g fat, 207kcal

Pitta Breads or Flatbreads

Either leave the bread plain and use as pitta or top with oil and za'atar or seeds and serve as flatbread.

MAKES 8

1 x quantity of dough (page 124)
2 tablespoons za'atar or 1 teaspoon
  cumin seeds (optional)

Preheat the oven to 220°C/200°C fan/425°F/gas mark 7 and line 1–2 trays with greased baking parchment. Make up your dough following the recipe for the Sesame Seed Buns (page 124).

Divide the dough into 8 balls and flatten onto the trays. You want to make ovals about 12 x 20cm (4½ x 8in) and ensure that they are not less than 5mm (¼in) thick, otherwise they won't fold to hold your fillings. To make flatbreads, brush over the oil and scatter over the za'atar or seeds. Cook for 10–12 minutes or until golden brown and firm to the touch. Remove from the tray and cool on a rack.

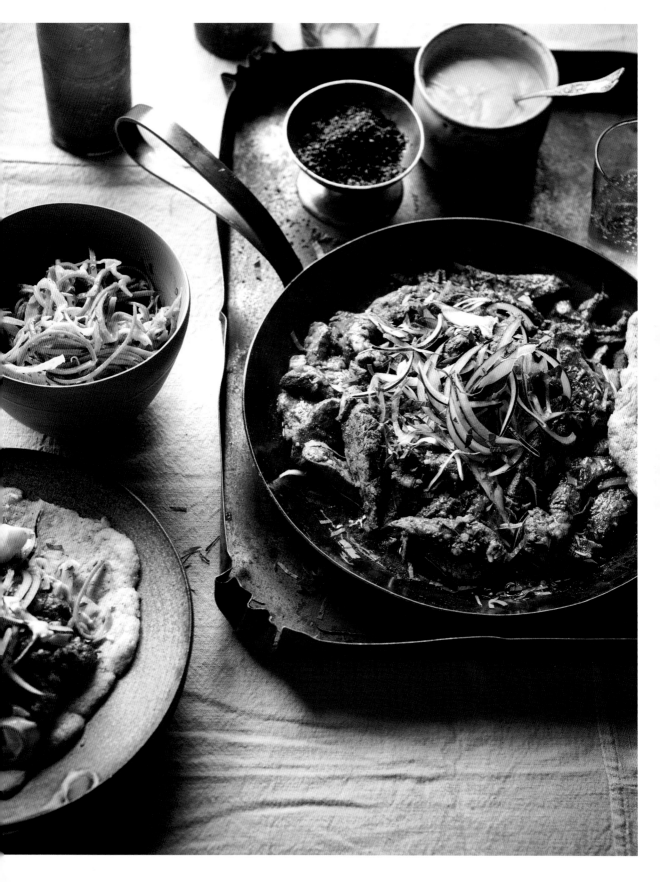

Flavio's Oven-baked Chips

Since potatoes are not part of a low-carb diet, we have come up with some even-better-than-spud alternatives, packed with colour and flavour. Try one on its own or a mixture together. Serve them up while they're hot with the Tomato Relish (page 123), Burger Relish (page 124) or the Peri-peri Dipping Sauce (page 112).

To give you some carb comparisons per 100g (3½oz): sweet and ordinary potatoes contain 17g net carbs, celeriac and okra have 7g, carrots 6.8g and swede, the lowest of all, has just 5.6g, so take your pick wisely at the greengrocers.

Preheat the oven to 220°C/200°C fan/425°F/gas mark 7. Line one or two baking trays with baking parchment.

Peel the root vegetables and cut into chips. Rinse the okra and dry with kitchen paper. Don't mix the two as they need different cooking times.

Toss the chips in a bowl with the oil and salt and ensure they are evenly coated. For spicy chips, make up the spice mixture and add to the oil and salt. Spread the chips out on the baking tray/s and cook the okra for about 15 minutes and the root vegetables for 20–25 minutes or until golden brown and crispy.

Once the chips are cooked, remove them from the oven and serve immediately.

SERVES 4

600g (1lb 5oz) celeriac, swede, carrot and/or okra
2 tablespoons extra virgin olive oil
salt

For the spicy chips
1 tablespoon smoked paprika
1 teaspoon cayenne pepper
2 teaspoons garlic powder

Per serving of root vegetable chips 6.9g carbs, 6.1g fibre, 2.5g protein, 7.4g fat, 116kcal
Per serving of okra chips 5.6g carbs, 7.9g fibre, 4.5g protein, 8.3g fat, 130kcal

Coleslaw

This is lovely to take to work, or to serve with the Southern-baked Chicken (page 115) or the Peri-peri Chicken (page 112), especially if you make your own mayonnaise (see page 78). You can replace the pumpkin seeds with peanuts, if you wish.

Dry–fry the seeds in a frying pan over a medium heat until lightly browned.

Combine the mayonnaise, vinegar, mustard, yogurt and seasoning together in a large mixing bowl. Season to taste, add the remaining ingredients and stir through to combine. Serve straight away or chill for up to a day before serving.

SERVES 6

50g (1¾oz) pumpkin seeds
150g (5½oz) mayonnaise (page 78)
2 tablespoons raw cider or white wine vinegar
2 tablespoons Dijon mustard
3 tablespoons Greek yogurt
150g (5½oz) sprouts or cabbage
300g (10½oz) red cabbage
1 large carrot, coarsely grated
1 apple, coarsely grated
3 spring onions, finely chopped
salt and freshly ground black pepper

Per serving 8.5g carbs, 3.2g fibre, 4.8g protein, 21g fat, 249kcal

Chinese Spare Ribs

Spare ribs offer economy, great flavour and the added joy of eating meat with your fingers. Usually this dish is laden with sugar but we have managed to make it equally tasty using the sweetness of the onion and a small amount of honey, reducing the carb load. Do ask your butcher to separate the meaty ribs for you or use a sharp cook's knife to cut between each one. The Chinese Green Stir-fry on page 119 makes the ideal partner for the ribs.

Preheat the oven to 200°C/180°C fan/400°F/gas mark 6.

Put the pork ribs into an ovenproof dish (like a lasagne dish) and season with salt and pepper. Pour warm water around the ribs so that they are half submerged. Cover the dish tightly with foil and cook for 1½ hours.

Meanwhile, make the sauce. Sweat the onion with the ginger and garlic in the olive oil in a saucepan over a medium heat for about 10 minutes. Don't let them burn; they should just soften slowly. Now add the remaining ingredients and stir through. Remove the pan from the heat.

Remove the dish from the oven and carefully peel away the foil, letting any steam out without scalding yourself. Check that the ribs are cooked through; the meat should fall easily from the bones. If they are not cooked through put them back into the oven for a little longer.

Remove the ribs from the dish and set aside on a warm plate. Pour the cooking liquid into a measuring jug (reserve the dish). Pour 150ml (¼ pint) into the saucepan with the sauce and return it to the heat. Bring to the boil, then simmer gently for 5 minutes. If the sauce is very thick, add a little more liquid until you have a pouring consistency. Discard any remaining liquid or keep to use as a stock.

Put the ribs back into the ovenproof dish and pour the sauce over, tossing them to make sure they are coated all over. Put the dish back into the oven for 30 minutes. Transfer to a serving plate, drizzle with the oil and scatter with the toasted sesame seeds and spring onions.

SERVES 6

1.2kg (3lb) pork ribs, separated
salt and freshly ground black pepper

For the sauce

1 onion, finely chopped
25g (1oz) ginger, grated
3 fat garlic cloves, grated
2 tablespoons extra virgin olive oil, pork fat or cold-pressed groundnut oil
2 teaspoons Chinese five-spice powder
½ teaspoon chilli flakes
3 tablespoons tamari or soy sauce
2 tablespoons Chinese rice vinegar or cider vinegar
2 teaspoons honey (optional)
2 teaspoons toasted sesame oil
2 teaspoons chilli powder
1 tablespoon tomato purée
4 tablespoons cold water

To serve

1 teaspoon toasted sesame oil
1 teaspoon toasted sesame seeds
3 spring onions, green and white parts, finely chopped

Per serving 6g carbs, 1.5g fibre, 40g protein, 29g fat, 448kcal

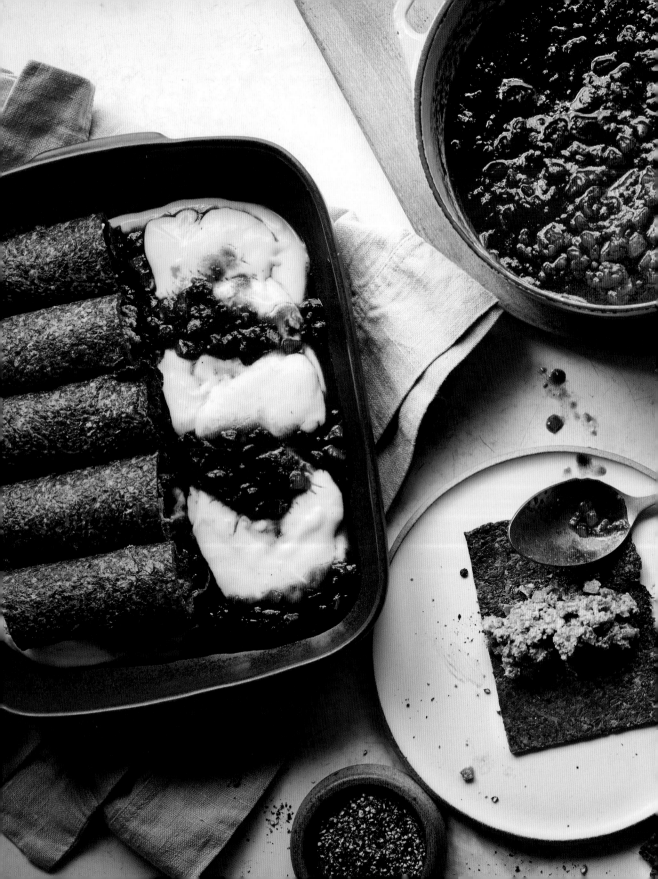

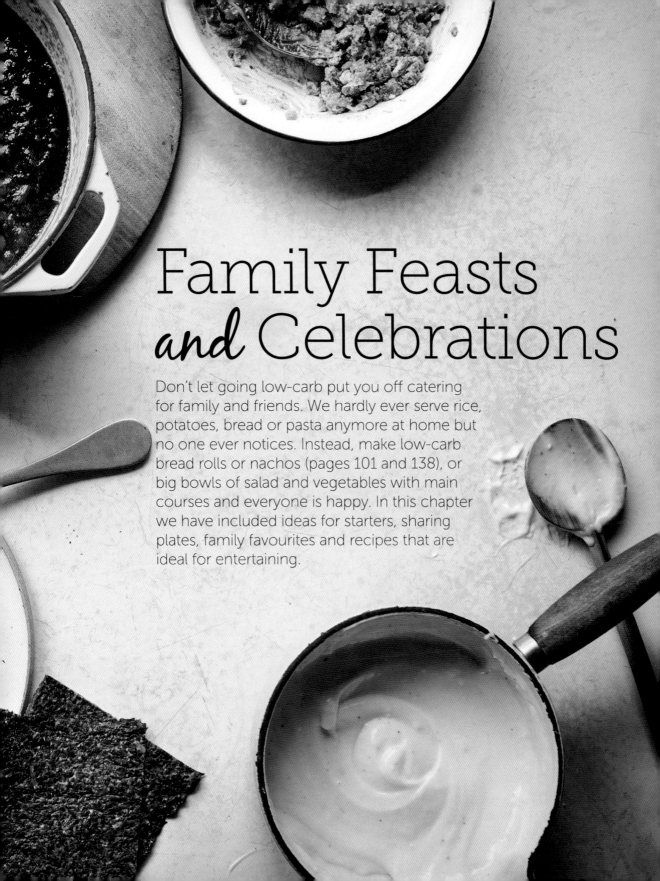

Family Feasts
and Celebrations

Don't let going low-carb put you off catering for family and friends. We hardly ever serve rice, potatoes, bread or pasta anymore at home but no one ever notices. Instead, make low-carb bread rolls or nachos (pages 101 and 138), or big bowls of salad and vegetables with main courses and everyone is happy. In this chapter we have included ideas for starters, sharing plates, family favourites and recipes that are ideal for entertaining.

Three Tomato, Burrata & Basil Salad

This stunning salad is perfect for entertaining or a quick supper with one of the low-carb rolls on page 101. The cherry tomatoes can be roasted a day earlier and stored in the fridge, but bring them to room temperature before serving. The fresh tomatoes can be cut and mixed, but wait to season them with salt or it will draw the water out.

Preheat the oven to 180°C/160°C fan/350°F/gas mark 4. Lay the cherry tomatoes, cut side up, on a baking tray and scatter with salt and pepper and two-thirds of the thyme sprigs. Roast for 30 minutes or until softened and starting to brown. Remove from the oven and set aside to cool.

Mix the sun-dried and fresh tomatoes together in a bowl. Season the oil with salt and pepper to taste and use half of it to dress the fresh tomatoes when you are about to serve. Arrange on a serving dish or a wooden board that has a groove around the edge to catch the juices.

Add the burrata and roasted tomatoes and finish with a flurry of basil leaves over the fresh tomatoes and the remaining thyme over the cheese. As you serve, cut the burrata in half and pour over the remaining seasoned olive oil.

SERVES 6

300g (10½oz) cherry tomatoes, halved
a small bunch of thyme
150g (5½oz) sun-dried tomatoes, drained and roughly chopped
600g (1lb 5oz) assorted fresh, ripe tomatoes, halved or cut into 3cm (1¼in) dice
4 tablespoons best extra virgin olive oil
a large handful of basil leaves
3 burrata or buffalo mozzarella, drained, approx. 400g (14oz) in total
salt and freshly ground black pepper

Per serving 7.7g carbs, 2.8g fibre, 23g protein, 47g fat, 559kcal

Low-carb Nachos

These were invented by a Mexican maître d'hôtel, Ignacio Anaya, whose nickname was "Nacho". Legend has it that he whipped up this dish for a group of hungry US military wives from a nearby base in 1943. They loved it, took the idea home with them and it spread. Our version has fewer carbs and sauces that aren't loaded with sugar.

Preheat the grill to hot. Spread the crackers in a single layer over a large heatproof plate. Scatter over the cheese and put under the grill until the cheese has just melted.

Remove from the oven and scatter over the tomatoes, chilli and coriander. Serve with Rose's sauce and Robbie's salsa dolloped on top or on the side.

SERVES 4

½ x quantity of Flaxseed Crackers (page 85)
150g (5½oz) mature Cheddar, coarsely grated
100g (3½oz) tomatoes, cubed
2 green chillies, finely sliced
a small bunch of coriander, leaves picked and stalks finely chopped

To serve
½ quantity of Rose's Green & Lovely Sauce (page 120)
½ quantity of Robbie's Hot Salsa Roja (page 122)

Per serving 11g carbs, 4.7g fibre, 19g protein, 48g fat, 568kcal

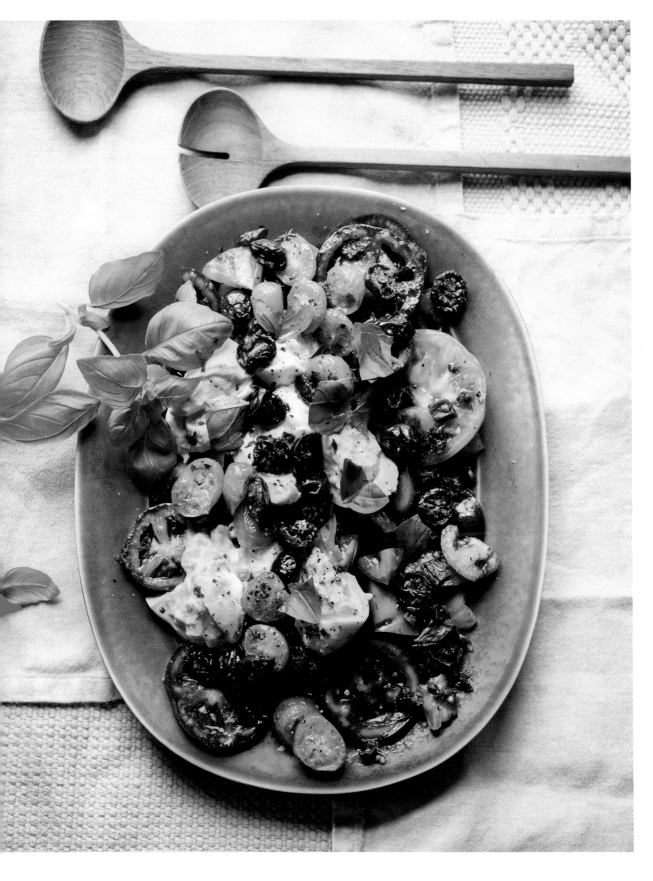

Lamb Shank Tagine

This is ideal entertaining food, as it can either be prepared in advance or it will sit patiently in the oven while you assemble the rest of the meal. It also freezes well. Saffron adds an earthy flavour and golden colour to the dish, but if you don't have it, leave it out. And if you are being very low-carb, leave the prunes out.

Preheat the oven to 170°C/150°C fan/340°F/gas mark 3½.

Season the lamb shanks with a teaspoon of salt. Heat the fat in a very large ovenproof saucepan or casserole dish and brown the lamb shanks. It will take around 30 minutes to get them really brown on all sides and on each flat end; keep turning them as each side browns. Use tongs to remove the shanks from the pan and set aside in another dish or bowl. If there is a lot of fat, pour most of this away, but leave enough in the pan to fry the vegetables.

Add the onion, garlic and leek to the same pan and sweat them over a medium heat for 7–10 minutes or until the vegetables are translucent. Return the lamb shanks to the casserole dish and add the remaining ingredients. Season with another teaspoon of salt and some pepper and bring to the boil. Push the lamb shanks under the surface of the liquid. Cover with a lid or tightly with foil (or transfer to a tagine)and cook in the oven for about 2½ hours or until the meat falls from the bone.

Scatter with the coriander sprigs and serve with the cauliflower couscous.

SERVES 6

6 lamb shanks, approx. 350–400g (12–14oz) each
4 tablespoons dripping, lard or extra virgin olive oil
1 onion, finely sliced into half moons
3 fat garlic cloves, lightly crushed
1 leek, finely chopped
6 prunes, pitted (optional)
2 teaspoons ground cumin
1 heaped teaspoon ground turmeric
1 heaped teaspoon ground cinnamon
1 teaspoon ground ginger
1 teaspoon saffron strands (optional)
2.5 litres (4½ pints) hot meat or chicken stock or hot water
salt and freshly ground black pepper

To serve

a few sprigs of coriander
pomegranate seeds
Orange & Harissa Cauliflower Couscous (page 67)

Per serving 5.8g carbs, 1.4g fibre, 50g protein, 32g fat, 515kcal

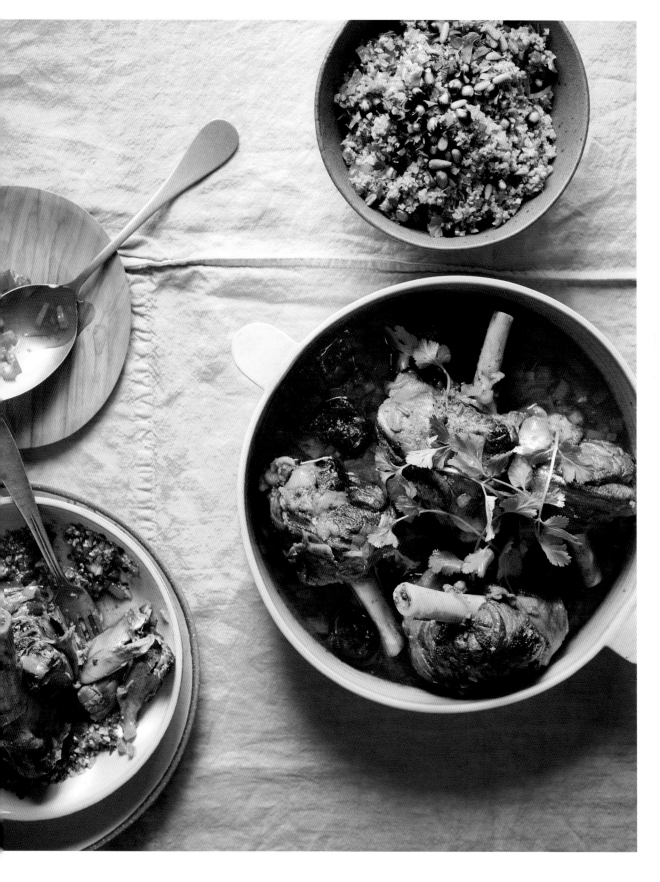

Pot-roast Chicken with Chorizo & Thyme

Smoky, garlicky chorizo is always popular in our household; we love the fact that a little gives instant colour and flavour to stews, soups, omelettes or vegetables. Any cut of chicken on the bone will work for this dish so, to reduce cost, legs are a good option; the long cooking time gets them gorgeously soft and tender. Do be fussy in your choice of olives; the flavour is so much better if you buy them with pits. Good-quality black Kalamata or Taggiasche are best here. To remove the pits, squash them with the flat blade of a knife and the pits will pop out.

Season the pieces of chicken with salt and pepper all over. Heat a large casserole or wide saucepan over a medium–high heat and brown the chicken, skin-side down first, thoroughly all over. The fat will come out of the chicken and the pieces will loosen from the pan. Let each piece become golden before turning it. They will take up to 30 minutes.

Remove the chicken from the pan and pour two-thirds of the fat into a dish; you can use this another day.

Put the pan back on the heat, add the onion and peppers and stir through. Cook for 5 minutes before adding the chorizo, two-thirds of the fresh thyme (or all of the dried thyme) and the garlic. Allow to cook for just a minute, then return the chicken pieces to the pan. Increase the heat so that they sizzle and pour in the wine; allow it to evaporate for 5 minutes, for the strong smell of alcohol to disappear, before adding the tomato purée, olives and stock. Bring the stew to the boil, then reduce the heat to a simmer.

Cover the pan, leaving the lid ajar to let out some of the liquid, or partially cover it with foil. Let the stew cook over a low heat for about 1 hour. Remove the lid or foil and check the meat – it should fall off the bone easily. Keep cooking for up to 30 minutes more if not. Stir in the cream, heat through and taste for seasoning, adjusting as necessary.

Scatter over the remaining fresh thyme and serve with low-carb bread rolls (see page 101), vegetable mash (see page 160) or green vegetables.

SERVES 6

1 large chicken, jointed, or 6 large chicken thighs, bone in and skin on (approx. 1.8kg/4lb in total)
½ teaspoon freshly ground black pepper
1 onion, coarsely sliced from root to tip
2 red or yellow peppers, each sliced into 10 lengths
50g (5½oz) chorizo, skinned and thinly sliced into circles
few sprigs of fresh thyme or 1 teaspoon dried thyme
3 garlic cloves, finely chopped
175ml (6fl oz) dry white wine
2 tablespoons tomato purée
12 good-quality black olives, pitted
300ml (½ pint) chicken or vegetable stock or hot water
75ml (2¾fl oz) double cream
salt

Per serving 7.7g carbs, 2.9g fibre, 58g protein, 30g fat, 545kcal

Cleopatra's Jamaican Curry Goat

I have been on a mission to find the perfect goat curry recipe since enjoying it some years ago. After tasting samples from Brixton, talking to my Jamaican friend Kwame Richardson and following Levi Roots' recipe, I met stylist to the stars Nicole Kerr, who was raised on curry goat cooked by her mother Cleopatra and father Constantine from Jamaica. This is based on Cleopatra's recipe with a few additions to achieve a delicious curry of tender meat, warmth and Caribbean spice. If you can't find goat, use mutton or lamb but cut the cooking time by an hour.

It is typical to add potatoes to the stew but I have swapped them for swede, which is so much lower in carbs. Jamaicans will tell you to use only Caribbean curry powder for an authentic flavour and to marinate the meat for 24 hours, but actually after 30 minutes no marinade can penetrate any further into meat, so we just suggest marinating it for 30 minutes. If you want to leave it for longer, then do, but it won't produce a better result.

For the marinade, cook the curry powder in the oil and butter in a saucepan for 2–3 minutes until it darkens slightly, then tip into a mixing bowl to cool for 10 minutes.

Put the meat into the bowl along with the rest of the marinade ingredients and stir through to ensure it is well combined. Cover and leave to marinate for 30 minutes, or up to overnight in the fridge.

To make the curry, put the oil and butter into a heavy-based pan over a medium-high heat. When hot, cook the meat until browned all over; it will take 15–20 minutes to do this thoroughly. Then add the tomato purée and 700ml (1¼ pints) of the hot stock, cover and cook for 2 hours over a low heat, stirring occasionally.

After this time, add all the remaining ingredients including the remaining 300–500ml (10–18fl oz) hot stock (enough to cover the vegetables) and continue to cook, uncovered, over a low heat for 30–40 minutes or until the meat and swede are tender. Keep an eye on the curry and add a little hot water to stop it drying out. Remove the Scotch bonnet if you don't want the heat or break it up and stir it in for a very spicy kick. Taste the stew for seasoning. Serve hot in bowls with low-carb bread rolls (page 101) or cauli-rice (page 66).

SERVES 8

1.5kg (3lb 5oz) lean goat or
    mutton, cubed
2 tablespoons extra virgin olive oil
30g (1oz) butter
2 tablespoons tomato purée
1–1.2 litres (1¾–2 pints) hot meat
    stock or water
1 medium onion, roughly
    chopped
4 sprigs of thyme
2 bay leaves
2 spring onions, roughly chopped
4 garlic cloves, lightly crushed
15g (½oz) ginger, peeled and
    grated
600g (1lb 5oz) swede, peeled and
    cut into bite-size pieces
1 Scotch bonnet chilli

For the marinade

5 tablespoons Caribbean mild
    curry powder
2 tablespoons extra virgin olive oil
30g (1oz) butter
1 teaspoon salt
1 teaspoon freshly ground black
    pepper
1 heaped teaspoon crushed
    allspice berries
4 cloves, crushed
1 tablespoon ground coriander
1 teaspoon ground cumin
2 tablespoons tamari or soy sauce

Per serving 8.3g carbs, 1.7g fibre, 54g protein, 38g fat, 598kcal

Mechoui Leg of Lamb

This Moroccan recipe is a great entertaining dish that can be prepared the day before. We love it with the crunchy all-colourful slaw based on a tabbouleh salad, labneh or Greek yogurt with fresh coriander.

Preheat the oven to 240°C/220°fan/475°F/gas mark 9. Remove the lamb from the fridge and allow to come to room temperature for 30 minutes.

Mix the ingredients for the spiced butter together in a bowl. Put the lamb onto a large oven tray or roasting dish and use a long, sharp-pointed knife to make about 7 incisions about 5cm (2in) deep. Push a little spiced butter into each cut, forcing it in as far as you can. Do the same on the other side. Season the lamb lightly and lay onto the tray over the sliced onions. Rub the remaining butter over the lamb.

Pour the cold water into the tray. Wrap it tightly in two layers of foil and roast for 10 minutes. Reduce the oven temperature to 180°C/160°C fan/350°F/gas mark 4 and roast for 3 hours. Remove the lamb from the oven, then carefully lift a corner of the foil and pull the bone away slightly. The meat around it should be tender and about to fall off the bone. If it is not, replace the foil and put the lamb back in the oven. When the lamb is cooked through, remove it from the tray and rest for 20 minutes with the foil and a tea towel on top to keep it warm.

Now take a look at the cooking juices left in the tray. If there is a lot of fat, skim most of this off. Heat the tray on the hob. If there isn't much liquid left, add 100–200ml (3½–7fl oz) hot water and stir through. Taste the juices and adjust the seasoning before pouring into a warm jug to serve.

SERVES 8

1 leg of lamb, approx. 2kg (4lb 8oz)
200ml (7fl oz) cold water
2 onions sliced into rings approx.
  1cm (½in) wide
250g (9oz) labneh or Greek yogurt
a handful of coriander leaves,
  stems chopped, to serve

For the spiced butter

100g (3½oz) butter, softened
1 teaspoon salt
½ teaspoon ground cloves
2 teaspoons smoked paprika
1 teaspoon ground cinnamon
1 teaspoon ground turmeric
2 teaspoons ground cumin
2 teaspoons hot chilli powder
½ teaspoon ground black pepper
25g (1oz) ginger, grated
5 garlic cloves, finely chopped

Per serving of lamb 5g carbs, 1g fibre, 73g protein, 49g fat, 754kcal

Tabbouleh Slaw

We love the bright colours and flavours of tabbouleh and have been taught to make it by our friend Amal. We replace the bulgur wheat with shredded red cabbage for volume, colour and crunch. I add in rocket if I am short of parsley.

SERVES 8

450g (1lb) red cabbage, finely shredded
4 spring onions, finely chopped
100g (3½oz) parsley, leaves roughly chopped, stalks finely chopped
a small handful of mint leaves
250g (9oz) tomatoes, diced
100g (3½oz) pomegranate seeds

For the dressing

juice of 2 large lemons
4 tablespoons extra virgin olive oil
1 tablespoon pomegranate molasses
  or 1 tablespoon balsamic vinegar and
  1 teaspoon honey
1 tablespoon sumac
1 small garlic clove, grated
1 tablespoon red wine vinegar
½ teaspoon salt and some freshly
  ground black pepper

Put the salad ingredients into a bowl and make the dressing by mixing the ingredients together. Combine the dressing and salad. Serve straight away or keep cool for up to an hour before serving.

Per serving 6.5g carbs, 2.9g fibre, 1.3g protein, 6.6g fat, 99kcal

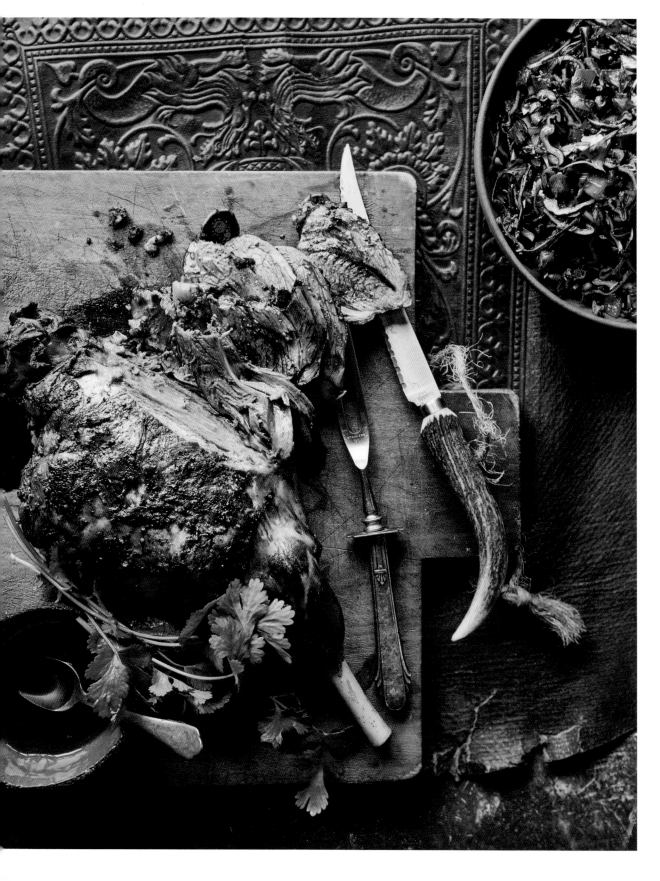

Spinch Pasta Cannelloni

Years ago when I was asked to prepare cannelloni for a group of keen-cooking Italian mamas, I could see them examining me and judging the English writer on her knowledge. When they asked for more, I realized I had passed the test and I have been making cannelloni ever since. See them being made on page 136.

To make the ragù, heat the oil in a pan over a low heat and fry the carrot, celery and onion with the garlic and rosemary for 15 minutes until soft.

Meanwhile, split the skins of the sausages and put the meat onto a chopping board. Discard the skins. Chop the meat finely with a large knife. British sausages contain starch that makes them sticky, whereas Italian sausages, which are all meat, crumble easily.

Add the sausage meat to the pan and brown well, bashing it with a wooden spoon to break it up. Allow any meat juices to evaporate before adding the wine and tomato purée. Cook the ragù for 15–25 minutes over a low heat or until the meat is cooked through, adding a little water if the sauce looks dry. The ragù is now ready to eat or to cool to use for cannelloni.

If you want a cheese filling, gently combine all the ingredients and use this instead instead of the ragù filling.

To make the béchamel, mix 3 tablespoons of the milk with the cornflour in a small bowl until smooth. Pour into a saucepan with the remaining sauce ingredients and put over a medium heat. Whisk to combine, once it has thickened and is bubbling remove from the heat. Season to taste.

Preheat the oven to 200°C/fan 180°C/400°F/gas mark 6.

Transfer the cooled ragù to a bowl and stir in the ricotta. If you have just cooked the spinach pasta sheets, leave them on the tray or spread them out onto a work surface to stuff them. Cut each sheet into 9 smaller rectangles measuring about 10 x 12cm (4 x 4½in). Divide the ragù mixture between the 18 rectangles, dolloping it into the centre of each one (see page 136). Spread the filling out a little, roll up each rectangle and set aside.

Drop spoonfuls of half the béchamel and half the tomato sauce on the base of a large ovenproof dish; you may need two dishes, as the cannelloni need a bit of space between each roll. Lay the rolls on top 2cm (¾in) apart and drop spoonfuls of the remaining two sauces on top. Scatter over the Parmesan and bake for 20–25 minutes or until bubbling hot throughout. Let the cannelloni settle for at least 10 minutes before enjoying.

SERVES 6 (3 cannelloni each)

2 sheets of Spinach Pasta
  (page 100)
½ quantity of Quick Italian Tomato
  Sauce (page 50)
25g (1oz) Parmesan or Grana
  Padano, finely grated
salt and freshly ground black
  pepper

For the sausage ragù

3 tablespoons extra virgin olive oil
1 small carrot, finely diced
1 celery stick, finely diced
1 small red onion, finely diced
2 garlic cloves, lightly crushed
1 sprig of rosemary
8 gluten-free, high meat-content
  pork sausages or Italian sausages
  approx. 400g (14oz) in total
5 tablespoons white wine
1 tablespoon tomato purée
100g (3½oz) ricotta

For a cheese filling

500g (1lb 2oz) ricotta
60g (2¼oz) soft herbs, such as a
  mixture of chives, parsley and basil
75g (2¾oz) Parmesan, finely grated
1 teaspoon freshly grated nutmeg

For the béchamel

550ml (19fl oz) whole milk
4 tablespoons cornflour
50g (1¾oz) butter
½ teaspoon salt
¼ teaspoon freshly grated nutmeg
1 bay leaf

Per serving (sausage filling)
23g carbs, 6.8g fibre, 57g protein,
66g fat, 720kcal
Per serving (cheese filling)
22g carbs, 6.3g fibre, 52g protein,
62g fat, 873kcal

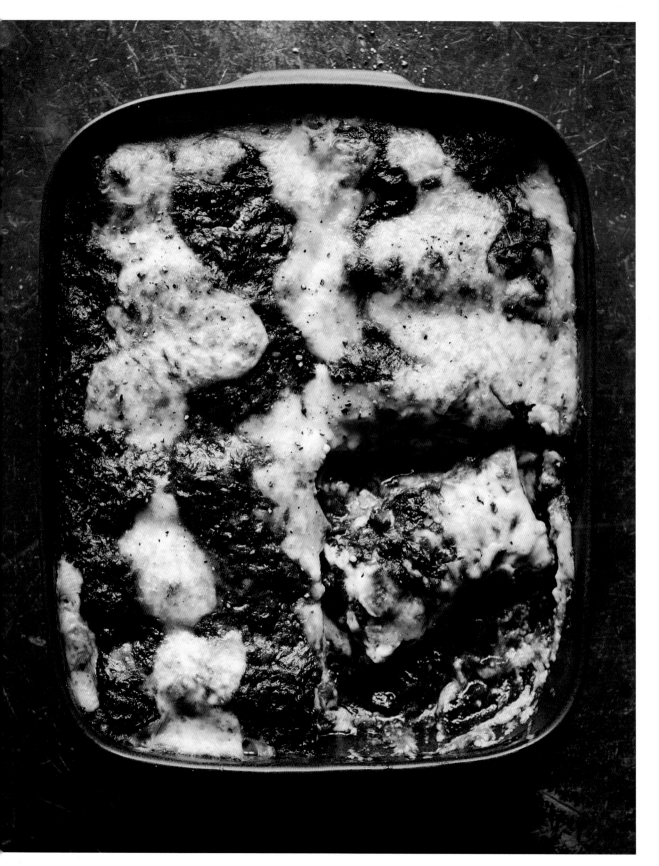

Roast Salmon with Sesame & Spring Onion Crust

This stunning salmon dish is easy to make; the onion curls and sesame seeds can be prepared in advance. Serve with the Chinese Green Stir-Fry (page 119), Cauli-Rice (page 66) or a Green Salad (page 78).

Preheat the oven to 200°C/180°C fan/400°F/gas mark 6. Cut the green parts off the spring onions and then slice them lengthways into strips, keeping one end intact. Put into a bowl filled with cold water to soak – they will curl. Cut the white parts diagonally and set aside. Toast the sesame seeds in a dry frying pan until golden brown, then set aside.

Put the salmon into a roasting dish. Brush with 1 tablespoon of the olive oil and scatter over salt and the pepper. Roast for 20 minutes or until firm to the touch and cooked through. Transfer to a serving plate and keep warm.

Heat the remaining olive oil and the sesame oil over a high heat and fry the chilli, white parts of the spring onions, garlic and ginger for just a few minutes until lightly golden. Stir in the tamari, and as soon as it bubbles, pour over the salmon and dress with the toasted sesame seeds. Drain the green spring onion curls, pull them apart and scatter alongside or over the salmon.

SERVES 6

8 spring onions
2 tablespoons sesame seeds
1 side of salmon, approx. 1kg (2lb 4oz)
3 tablespoons extra virgin olive oil
1 teaspoon Szechuan or black peppercorns, crushed
1 teaspoon toasted sesame oil
1 hot red chilli, finely sliced on the diagonal
2 fat garlic cloves, finely sliced
10g (¼oz) ginger, peeled and julienned
2 tablespoons tamari or soy sauce
salt

Per serving 1.9g carbs, 0.8g fibre, 40g protein, 30g fat, 438kcal

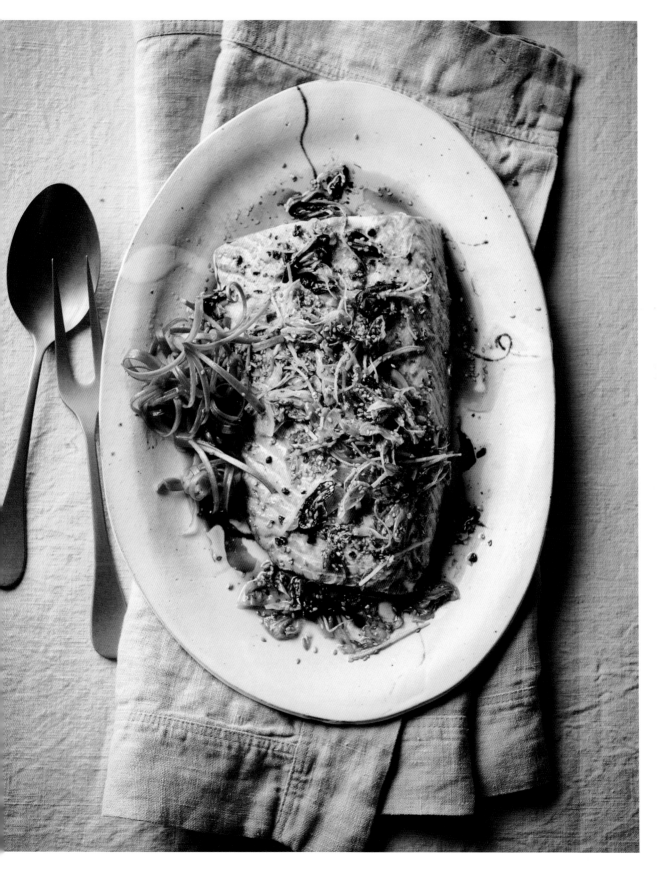

Toad in the Hole & Onion Gravy

This was one of my favourite home-cooked meals as a child. I loved to watch it rise in the oven, wrapping the sausages in a puffy duvet of savoury batter. Do seek out sausages made from all meat or with very little rusk or maize starch, as the carbs will be lower.

Make the batter by beating all the ingredients together with a whisk in a mixing bowl or whizz them briefly in a food processor. Leave the batter to rest while you cook the sausages. Preheat the oven to 240°C/220°C fan/475°F/gas mark 9. Put the sausages and fat into an ovenproof dish measuring about 20 x 30cm (8 x 12in) and cook for 20 minutes. Remove from the oven and pour in the batter straight away – it should sizzle as it goes in. Scatter over the thyme, if using.

Put the dish back in the oven for a further 15 minutes or until the batter is well risen, firm to the touch and a rich golden brown. Remove the dish from the oven and leave for a couple of minutes before serving.

SERVES 4

8 gluten-free pork sausages
3 tablespoons beef dripping, chicken fat, lard or olive oil
leaves from a few sprigs of thyme (optional)

For the batter
3 eggs
300ml (½ pint) whole milk
75g (2¾oz) chickpea (gram) flour
a good pinch of salt

Per serving 16g carbs, 2.7g fibre, 32g protein, 47g fat, 627kcal

Yorkshire Puddings

These can be cooked quickly in the fat and juices from roast meat while it rests.

MAKES 8 INDIVIDUAL YORKIES

3 tablespoons beef dripping, chicken fat, lard, or olive oil

For the batter
1 large egg
100ml (3½fl oz) whole milk
25g (1oz) chickpea (gram) flour
a good pinch of salt
a few thyme leaves (optional)
1 teaspoon English mustard powder (optional)

Preheat the oven to 240°C/220°C fan/475°F/ gas mark 9. Whisk the ingredients together for the batter.

Divide the fat between 8 holes of one or two non-stick Yorkshire pudding trays and put in the oven to heat for 5 minutes.

Remove the tray(s) and pour in the batter. Return the tray(s) to the oven and bake for 12 minutes or until the Yorkies are risen and golden brown.

Remove and allow to cool for a couple of minutes before turning out and serving.

Per serving 2.2g carbs, 0.5g fibre, 2.1g protein, 6.6g fat, 78kcal

Onion Gravy

This delicious, easy-to-prepare gravy doesn't need meat stock, so it is ideal for vegetarians.

SERVES 6
1 tablespoon exta virgin olive oil
50g (1¾oz) butter
1 white onion, thinly sliced
a few sprigs of thyme
200ml (7fl oz) white wine
1 tablespoon balsamic vinegar
300ml (½ pint) hot water or chicken stock
2 teaspoons cornflour
salt and freshly ground black pepper

Heat the oil and butter in a small saucepan and fry the onion with some seasoning and the thyme over a medium heat for around 15 minutes until softened and lightly browned. Add the wine and let it evaporate for about 5 minutes. Add the balsamic vinegar and the water and bring it to the boil again. Reduce the heat and let it simmer for about 20 minutes.

Mix the cornflour with a teaspoon of water, stir into the gravy and simmer until thickened. Season to taste and serve warm.

Per serving 4.3g carbs, 0.6g fibre, 0.5g protein, 9g fat, 115kcal

Georgian Stuffed Aubergines

Normally, these are made with sliced aubergines that are rolled or folded, but they can be dry and we love the look and the softness of roast aubergine halves, plus they are a lot less fiddly to make. The Georgians use blue fenugreek, which is harder to find, so we use fenugreek seeds, as these are easily available in supermarkets. Fenugreek is often used in curry, so it won't be a redundant spice at the back of your cupboard for long. These are lovely as a vegan dish in a buffet, hence the recipe serves 8, but as a main course you might want two each. They go well with the Mechoui Leg of Lamb (page 144) or the Green Salad with Lemon & Honey Dressing (pages 78–79).

Preheat the oven to 200°C/180°C fan/400°F/gas mark 6. Halve the aubergines lengthways. Make criss-cross shallow cuts in the surface of each half and lay them on a baking tray. Brush with olive oil and season with salt and pepper. Put into the oven to bake for 45 minutes–1 hour. Remove from the oven when the aubergines are soft and push the centres down with a metal spoon to create cavities to stuff with the filling.

While the aubergines are cooking, make the filling by whizzing the walnuts, garlic, coriander, fenugreek, vinegar, salt and pepper together in a food processor, then gradually add the hot water to form a rough paste. Alternatively, use a pestle and mortar to crush the walnuts, garlic, coriander and fenugreek together before adding the vinegar and water. Taste and adjust the seasoning.

Spoon the filling into the cavities of the aubergines and flatten off with the back of the spoon. Pile the tomatoes on top of each one and put the tray back into the oven for 15 minutes or until the tomato has just softened. Remove from the oven and serve straight away, scattered with the herbs.

SERVES 8

3 aubergines
2 tablespoons extra virgin olive oil, to brush
200g (7oz) walnuts
3 garlic cloves
2 teaspoons ground coriander
1½ teaspoons fenugreek seeds, ground
4 teaspoons white wine vinegar
150ml (¼ pint) hot water
200g (7oz) tomatoes, diced
a handful of coriander or parsley leaves or dill fronds, to serve
salt and freshly ground black pepper

Per serving 4.5g carbs, 4.3g fibre, 5.7g protein, 21g fat, 237kcal

Chicken Parmigiana

This American-Sicilian classic dish was originally made with aubergines by the poor while the wealthy had the same dish made with meat. The aubergine recipe made its way to America with Italian immigrants after the Second World War and as they prospered, it was replaced with chicken or veal. Normally, it is made with breadcrumbs but we have swapped them for ground almonds.

Preheat the oven to 200°C/180°C fan/400°F/gas mark 6. Line a baking tray with baking parchment.

Cut the chicken breasts in half along the side and open them up like a book. Cut through the spine of each 'book' so that you have two separate halves. Place the halves between two pieces of heavy-duty plastic and pound the chicken breasts with a meat tenderizer or the base of a small saucepan until around 5mm (¼in) thick. Peel off the plastic, season with salt and pepper and scatter half the oregano over the chicken, pressing it in with your hands. Turn the flattened chicken breasts over and season the other side.

Prepare three shallow bowls: one with the flour, one with the beaten eggs and one with the ground almonds mixed with half the Parmesan. Dip the chicken pieces first in the flour, shaking off any excess, then in the egg and then the almond crumbs, making sure they are evenly coated. Lay the chicken on the prepared tray and brush lightly with the oil. Put into the oven for 15 minutes, then remove from the oven and set aside.

Pour a thin layer of the tomato sauce into a large ovenproof dish and lay the chicken pieces in the dish. Spoon a heaped tablespoon of sauce over each piece. Arrange the mozzarella on top of the chicken and scatter over the remaining oregano and Parmesan. Bake in the oven for 10 minutes or until the cheese is melted and the chicken is cooked through (make sure there are no pink juices when you pierce the thickest part with a skewer or the internal temperature is 85°C/185°F when measured with a probe thermometer). Remove from the oven and serve straight away, scattered with the basil.

SERVES 6

4 boneless, skinless chicken breasts, approx. 800g (1lb 12oz) in total
2 teaspoons dried oregano, plus extra to sprinkle
50g (1½oz) chickpea (gram) flour
2 eggs, beaten
150g (5½oz) ground almonds
75g (2¾oz) Parmesan, finely grated
2 tablespoons extra virgin olive oil
½ quantity of Quick Italian Tomato Sauce (page 50)
2 x 125g (4½oz) balls of mozzarella, cut into slices 1cm (½in) thick and drained in a sieve
salt and freshly ground black pepper
a few basil leaves, to serve

Per serving 8.7g carbs, 4.9g fibre, 63g protein, 42g fat, 677kcal

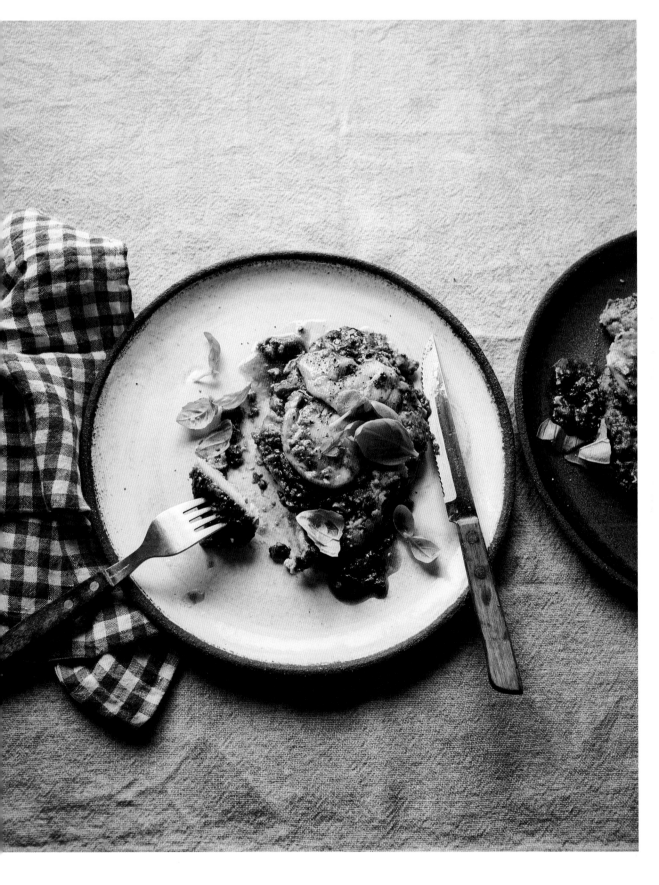

Pissaladière

This wonderfully flavourful dish comes from Nice in the south of France and is closely related to pizza from neighbouring Italy. It is perfect cut into squares while still warm and served with a crisp dry white wine. It can also be made in advance and reheated. If anchovies aren't your thing, do leave them off.

Preheat the oven to 200°C/180°C fan/400°F/gas mark 6. Line a 35 x 25cm (14 x 10in) baking tray with baking parchment and lightly brush it with olive oil.

Heat 2 tablespoons of the oil and the butter in a large frying pan over a low-medium heat. Add the onions, garlic, a small pinch of salt, some pepper, a few sprigs of thyme and the water and cook for 30–40 minutes; don't allow the onions to take any colour, just soften slowly. Remove from the heat and set aside to cool to room temperature.

Meanwhile, prepare the dough following the recipe on page 101.

Put the dough on the prepared baking tray and, with lightly oiled hands, start to flatten it. Pour over the remaining tablespoon of oil and flatten the dough with your fingers right to the edges. Bake in the oven for 10 minutes or just until it feels firm to the touch, but don't let it brown.

Squash the garlic cloves, if you can still see them, and stir in with the onions. Spread the onions evenly over the dough. Pick out the cooked thyme. Dress the pissaladière with the anchovies in lines diagonally across the bread to form a cross-hatch pattern. Dot each diamond shape with an olive. Scatter over the capers and remaining thyme. Drizzle over some more oil and bake for 15–20 minutes or until lightly browned.

SERVES 8
For the dough
1 quantity Flaxseed Bread Roll dough recipe (page 101)

For the topping
3 tablespoons extra virgin olive oil, plus extra to drizzle
25g (1oz) butter
750g (1lb 10oz) white or red onions, finely sliced
3 garlic cloves, lightly crushed
a small bunch of thyme
4 tablespoons water
20 anchovy fillets in oil, any larger fillets torn in half lengthways
about 25 black olives, pitted
1 tablespoon small capers, drained
salt and freshly ground black pepper

Per serving 9.4g carbs, 7.2g fibre, 14g protein, 28g fat, 357kcal

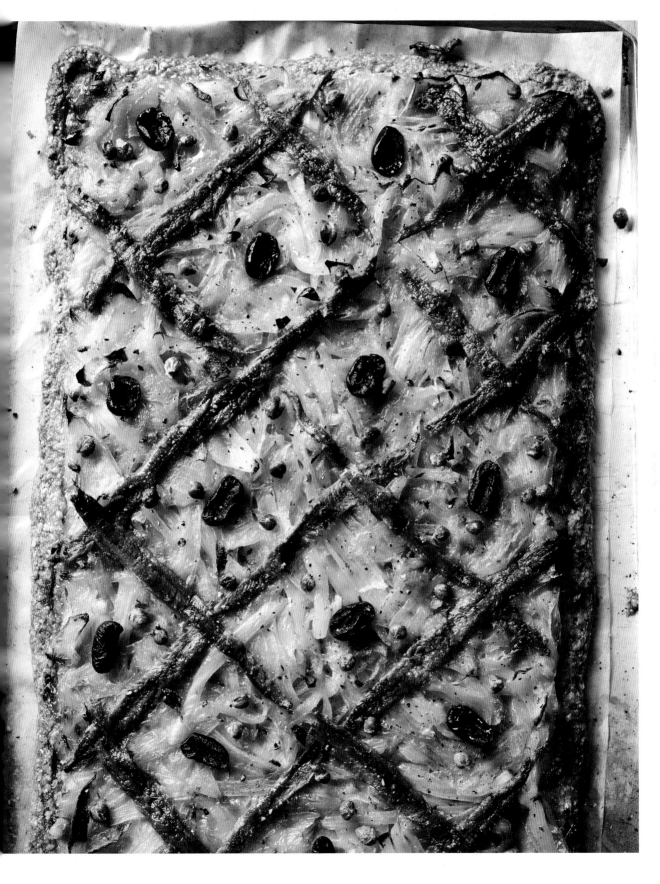

Kedgeree

This is easy and quick to make, and works well as a brunch or family supper, or in larger quantities for entertaining. I love the bright colours and warming flavours of the smoked fish and curry spices.

Poach the fish in the hot water in a saucepan for about 5 minutes or until cooked through. Remove the fish with a slotted spoon and leave to cool on a plate. Reserve the cooking water. When the fish is cool enough to touch, flake it into bite-size pieces.

Heat the oil and butter in a large frying pan and fry the onion and chilli, if using, for about 5 minutes over a medium heat until soft. Add the cauliflower with 200ml (7fl oz) of the reserved cooking water and stir through. Add the spices and stir again, put the lid on and leave to cook for 4 minutes. Stir in the fish and taste, seasoning with salt and pepper if needed. Cover for 2 minutes, then serve dotted with extra butter, the boiled egg quarters and herbs.

SERVES 4

500ml (18fl oz) hot water
250g (9oz) skinless smoked undyed haddock or other fish fillet
2 tablespoons extra virgin olive oil
50g (1¾oz) butter, plus a little extra to dot on top
1 onion, finely chopped
½–1 red or green chilli, finely sliced (optional)
1 small cauliflower and leaves (approx. 500g/1lb 2oz), riced (see page 66)
1 teaspoon ground turmeric
1 teaspoon ground coriander
2 teaspoons masala curry powder
4 hard-boiled eggs, quartered
a handful of parsley or coriander leaves, stalks finely chopped
salt and freshly ground black pepper

Per serving 12g carbs, 2.9g fibre, 15g protein, 17g fat, 264kcal

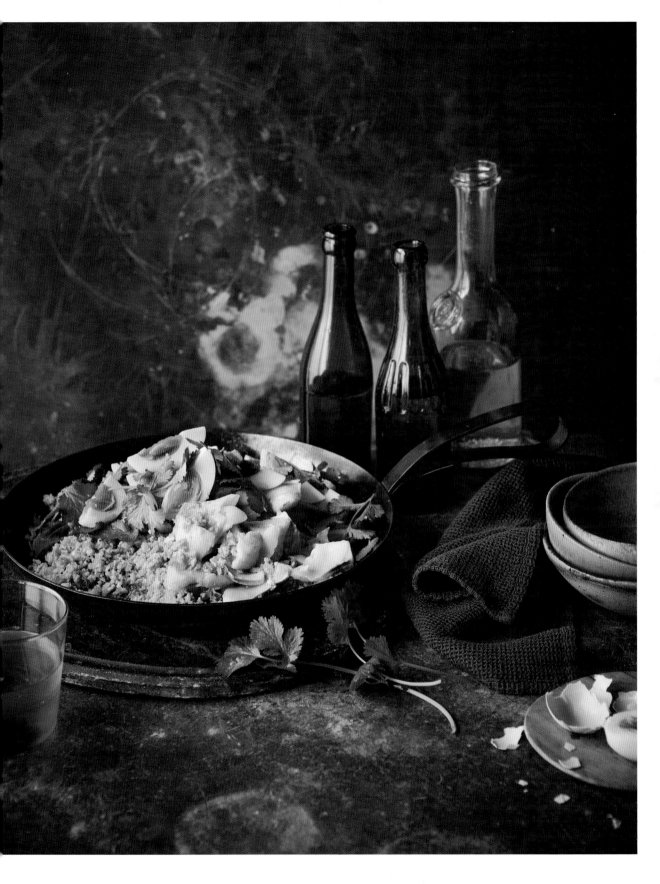

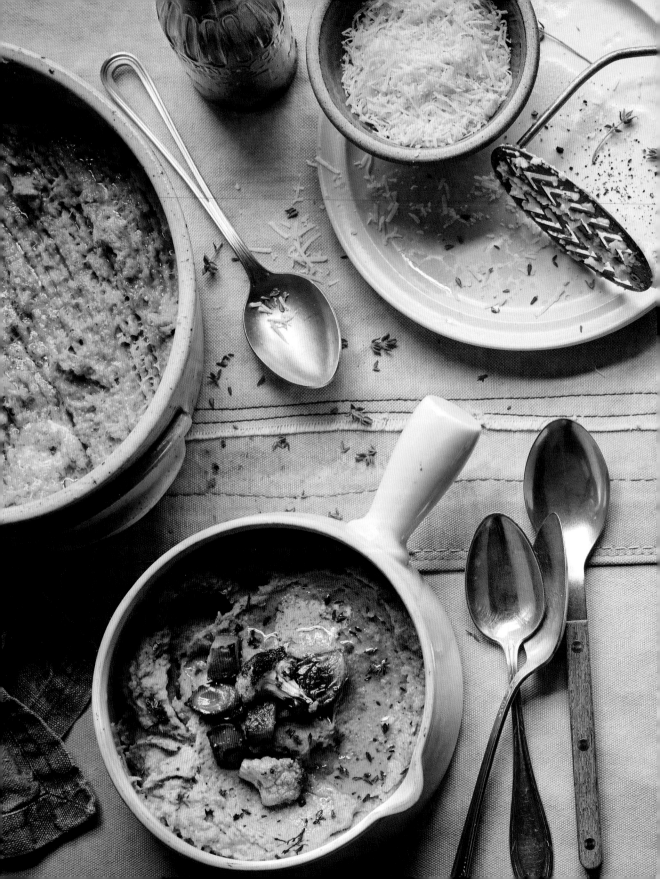

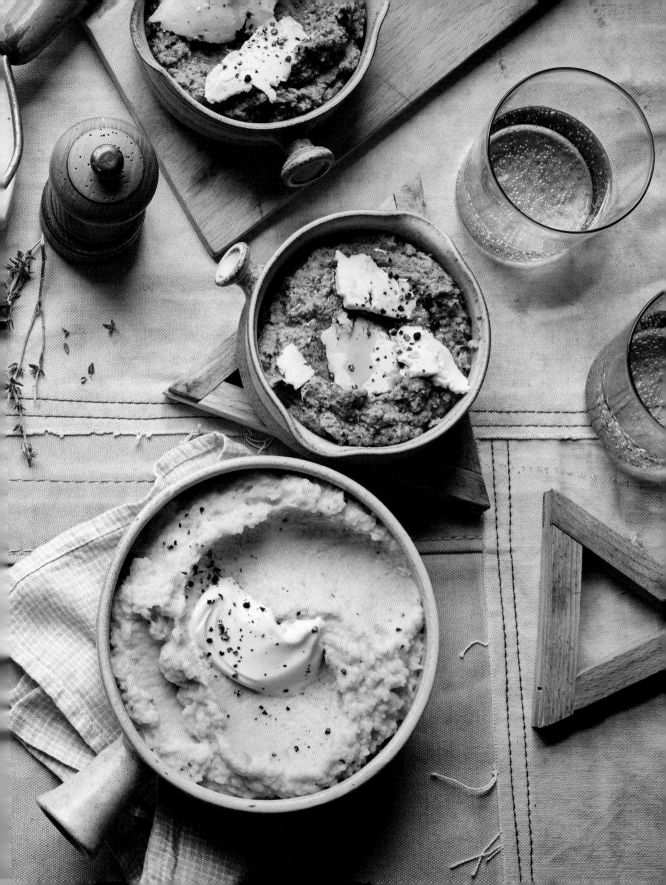

4 ways with... VEGETABLE MASH

Root vegetables, brassicas and squashes that aren't high in carbs are perfect for making a delicious rainbow of mash – with a fraction of the carbs of potato. Celeriac mash, for example, contains 4g ($^1/_8$oz) carbs per serving compared with potato mash at 24g (1oz). Celeriac is good with meat as well as fish, while cauliflower, sprouts and swede are better with meat, sausages and eggs. Pumpkin is also good, but butternut squash and parsnip could be used in moderation.

Vegetable mash can be made with a potato masher, but a food processor or stick blender gives the creamy texture that we all love. Any leftovers keep well in the fridge and make a good base for eggs the next day.

By using the leaves and stalk of the brassicas, you get a lot more mash. Cut the stalks into smaller pieces and cook first. Add the leaves last to ensure even cooking. Keep the mash plain or flavour with any of the suggestions below.

Basic Vegetable Mash

This recipe works for all vegetables, but as some are more absorbent than others, you will have to alter the milk quantity. In the photo on pages 158–159, it is made with swede and crème fraîche and is shown bottom right.

Steam or boil the vegetables until just tender. Drain well. Blend with the remaining ingredients in a food processor or with a stick blender until you have a soft, smooth mash. Taste and adjust the seasoning as necessary. Spoon into a warm bowl and dot with butter or add a dollop of crème fraîche to serve. (For nutritional info, see panel opposite.)

SERVES 4
400g (14oz) low-carb vegetable/s, such as cauliflower, celeriac, pumpkin, swede, Brussels sprouts or broccoli
25g (1oz) salted butter or extra virgin olive oil, plus extra to serve
25–75ml (1–2½fl oz) cow's milk, cream or crème fraîche, plus extra to serve
salt and freshly ground black pepper
½ teaspoon ground nutmeg (optional)

Cheesy Bubble & Squeak Mash

This recipe replaces normal bubble and squeak made with potato, which is therefore high in carbs. It is ideal for using up leftover sprouts or other vegetables instead. The portions are small, as it is filling. In the photo on pages 158–159 it is pictured top left.

Sauté the onion, garlic and chilli in the olive oil with seasoning in a frying pan over a medium heat until soft. Mix into the vegetable mash with three-quarters of the grated cheese. Spoon it into an ovenproof dish about 15 x 15cm (6 x 6in). Use a fork or a spoon to flatten it. Fleck the butter on top, scatter over the remaining cheese and bake in the oven at 200°C/180°C fan/400°F/gas mark 6 for 20 minutes or until piping hot.

SERVES 6
1 onion, finely chopped
1 fat garlic clove, finely chopped
a pinch of chilli flakes (optional)
2 tablespoons extra virgin olive oil
1 quantity of Basic Vegetable Mash made with sprouts (above)
75g (2½oz) Parmesan or Grana Padano, finely grated
10g (¼oz) salted butter
salt and freshly ground black pepper

Per serving 5.3g carbs, 2.4g fibre, 7.2g protein, 14g fat, 180kcal

Roast Vegetable Mash

This autumn-coloured, flecked mash is a triumph. Choose from a balance of low- to medium-carb vegetables; cauliflower keeps the carbs low, but squash and carrot give natural sweetness and colour. In the photo on pages 158–159 it is pictured bottom left.

Preheat the oven to 220°C/200°C fan/425°F/gas mark 7. Toss the harder vegetables, such as carrots, turnips, swede, celeriac and squash, in a mixing bowl with the thyme sprigs, garlic, half the olive oil and seasoning to coat. Spread them evenly on a baking tray and roast for 15 minutes. Then do the same with the remaining softer vegetables, such as the leeks, cauliflower, onions and radishes, and remaining oil and add them to the tray. Roast for a further 15 minutes or until all the vegetables are tender.

Squeeze the garlic from their skins into a food processor with the roasted veg and any oil from the tray. Whizz until flecked but not completely one colour (unless you prefer it that way). Serve straight away or reheat later. If it firms up too much for your liking, add a little milk or cream to let it down.

SERVES 6

1kg (2lb 4oz) mixed vegetables, such as pumpkin, cauliflower, celeriac, butternut squash, turnips, radishes, onions, leeks, carrots and swede
a few sprigs of thyme
6 tablespoons extra virgin olive oil
3 garlic cloves, unpeeled and lightly crushed
salt and freshly ground black pepper

Per serving 17g carbs, 2.7g fibre, 2.2g protein, 15g fat, 217kcal

Broccoli, Lemon & Thyme Mash with Feta

The flavours of lemon, thyme and feta give a Mediterranean feel to this mash. It is gorgeous with fish, sausages or roast meat. In the photo on pages 158–159 it is pictured top right.

Mix the grated feta, lemon zest and thyme into the hot vegetable mash. Season to taste and serve with the feta shavings and pepper on top.

SERVES 4

1 quantity of Basic Vegetable Mash made with broccoli (opposite)
75g (2½oz) feta, grated, plus 25g (1oz) shaved
1 teaspoon finely grated lemon zest
1 tablespoon thyme leaves
salt and freshly ground black pepper

Per serving 3.9g carbs, 2.8g fibre, 6.6g protein, 9.9g fat, 136kcal

Variations

Here are some further ideas for flavouring the mash.

- 1 heaped teaspoon mustard powder or Dijon mustard

- 1–2 tablespoons horseradish sauce, to taste

- 1 tablespoon thyme leaves, plus a few sprigs to serve

- 1 teaspoon cumin seeds

- 2 tablespoons fried bacon lardons

- 1 heaped tablespoon finely chopped chives

Per serving (sprout mash)
4.1g carbs, 2.6g fibre, 3.3g protein, 6.9g fat, 97kcal

Per serving (cauli mash)
4.1g carbs, 1.9g fibre, 2.4g protein, 6.5g fat, 88kcal

Per serving (swede mash)
2.9g carbs, 0.7g fibre, 0.8g protein, 5.7g fat, 67kcal

Per serving (pumpkin mash)
2.5g carbs, 0.5g fibre, 1.1g protein, 5.9g fat, 68kcal

Per serving (celeriac mash)
]3.2g carbs, 3.7g fibre, 1.9g protein, 6.2g fat, 84kcal

Per serving (broccoli mash)
2.4g carbs, 1.9g fibre, 2.5g protein, 5.4g fat, 72kcal

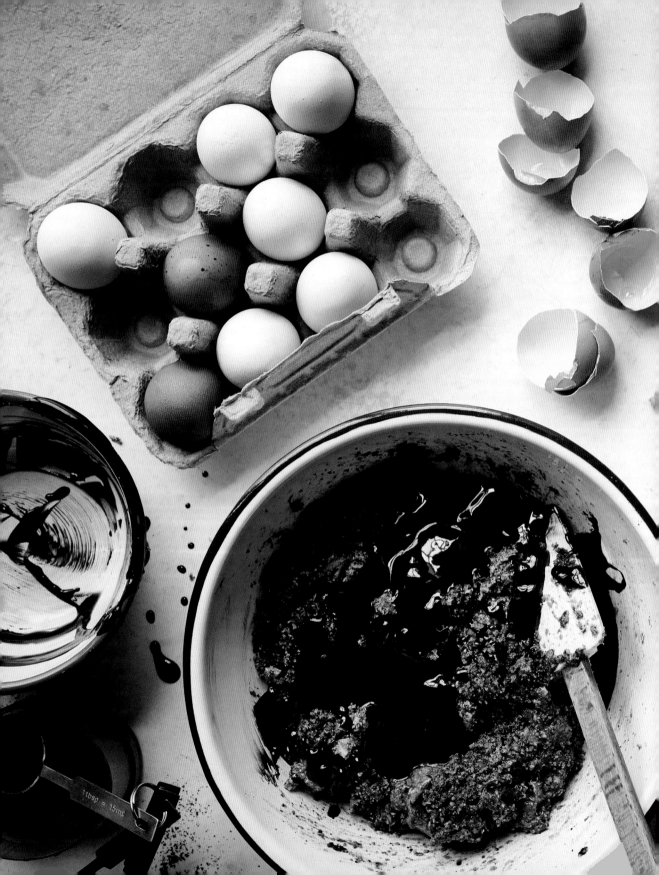

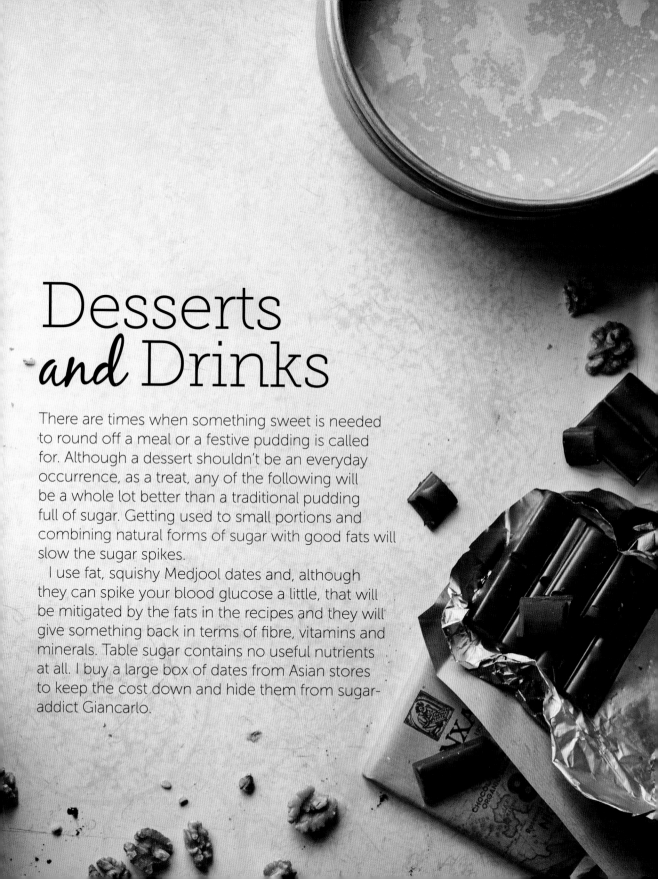

Desserts
and Drinks

There are times when something sweet is needed to round off a meal or a festive pudding is called for. Although a dessert shouldn't be an everyday occurrence, as a treat, any of the following will be a whole lot better than a traditional pudding full of sugar. Getting used to small portions and combining natural forms of sugar with good fats will slow the sugar spikes.

I use fat, squishy Medjool dates and, although they can spike your blood glucose a little, that will be mitigated by the fats in the recipes and they will give something back in terms of fibre, vitamins and minerals. Table sugar contains no useful nutrients at all. I buy a large box of dates from Asian stores to keep the cost down and hide them from sugar-addict Giancarlo.

Lemon Semifreddo

This delivers the soft Italian ice-cream experience without the sugar overload. We serve it in small portions with strawberries, blueberries, raspberries, blackberries or redcurrants and/or the Raspberry Sauce on page 176.

Line a 21 x 12 x 7cm (8¼ x 4½ x 2¾in) loaf tin with baking parchment, leaving the two long sides flapping over the edge. The excess can be used to cover the semifreddo while in the freezer and also for removing it later.

Soften the dates in the very hot water in a mug or small bowl. Mash them to a pulp with a fork and then push them through a sieve into a mixing bowl with the back of a spoon. Try to get as much purée from them as possible, discarding only the skins. Mix the date purée with the lemon zest and mascarpone.

Whisk the whipping cream in the large bowl of an electric mixer or by hand with a whisk. Add a little of this to the date and lemon zest mixture to loosen it, then fold the two together.

In a clean bowl, use a clean whisk or electric beaters to whisk the egg whites until they form stiff peaks. Take a little of this mixture and fold it gently into the whipped cream mixture to loosen it. Now gently fold in the rest, trying to keep the lightness and air in it. When it is just combined (don't overmix it), spoon it into the prepared tin, level the surface and cover with the flaps of baking parchment. Put it into the freezer for at least 8 hours.

Take the semifreddo out of the freezer 30 minutes before you wish to serve. Invert the semifreddo onto a chilled serving plate and peel away the paper. Serve whole, decorated with berries, or plated in slices, scattered with berries or with some Raspberry Sauce.

SERVES 8

4 Medjool dates, pitted
3 tablespoons very hot water
finely grated zest of 2 large
  lemons
150g (5½oz) mascarpone
150ml (¼ pint) whipping cream
3 egg whites
fresh berries or Raspberry Sauce
  (page 176), to serve (optional)

Per serving 10g carbs, 0.8g fibre, 2.7g protein, 16g fat, 198kcal

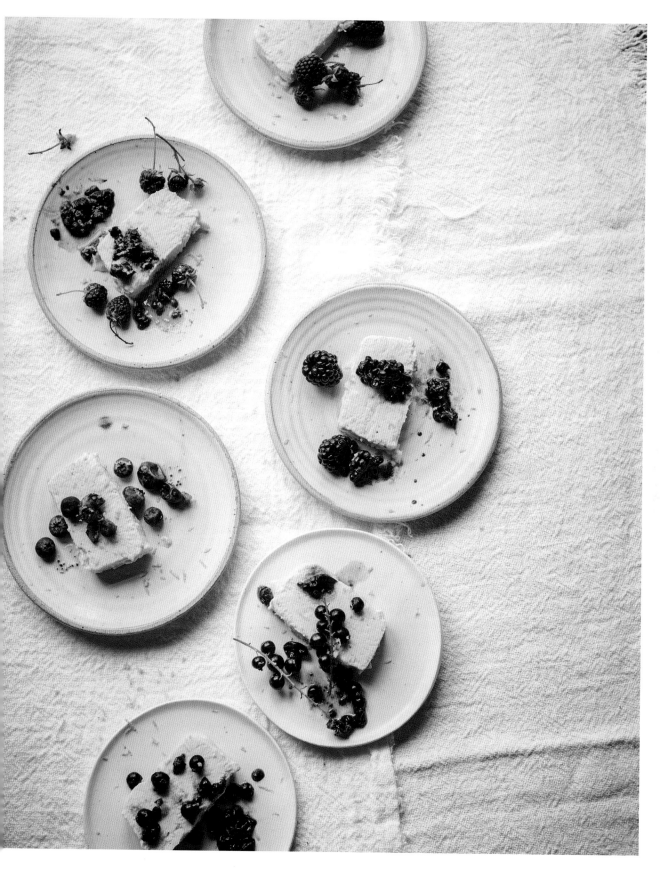

Baked Apricots with Walnut Stuffing & Vanilla Cinnamon Yogurt

Cooking late-autumn stone fruit brings out their jammy, naturally sweet flavours, and the simple walnut stuffing and whipped spiced yogurt transforms plums or apricots into an elegant dessert. Our recipe is based on cooking small ripe plums and apricots from room temperature. If your fruit are larger or less ripe, cover the dish with foil and cook for 20 minutes, then remove the foil and cook them, uncovered, for a further 30 minutes or until soft.

Preheat the oven to 200°C/180°C fan/400°F/gas mark 6. To make the stuffing, soften the dates in the very hot water and mash them to a purée with a fork. Mix the date purée with the remaining ingredients (apart from the fruit) in a small bowl. Lay the plum halves, cut side up, in an ovenproof dish. Use two teaspoons to fill the stone cavities with the stuffing. Put the dish into the oven for 25–30 minutes or until the stuffing is lightly browned and the fruit is just soft.

Meanwhile, make up the vanilla cinnamon yogurt by stirring the ingredients together in a small bowl. Taste and add honey, if you like. Serve chilled with the warm roasted fruits.

SERVES 6
2 Medjool dates, pitted
2 tablespoons very hot water
1 tablespoon softened butter
75g (2¾oz) walnuts, roughly chopped
1 teaspoon vanilla extract
9 plums or apricots, halved and stoned

For the vanilla cinnamon yogurt
250g (9oz) Greek yogurt
1 teaspoon ground cinnamon
2 teaspoons vanilla extract
1 teaspoon honey (optional)

Per serving 22g carbs, 3.8g fibre, 5.3g protein, 15g fat, 251kcal

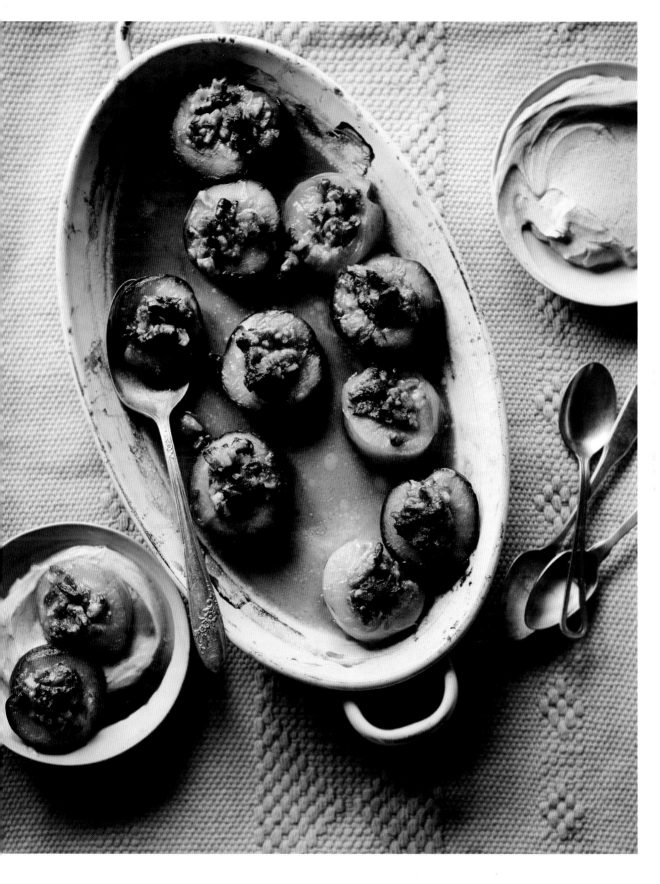

Baked Apples with Vanilla Custard

It seems everyone remembers their mother or grandmother baking apples, but the dish fell out of fashion. Since cooked apple is good for your gut health too there is every reason to have one when it's apple season. We have given two stuffing options here; as they are both so good, we couldn't choose between them.

To reduce the carb count of the custard by 3g, use almond milk, as it doesn't contain the milk sugar lactose. If you can't eat egg, you can use ready-made sugar-free custard powder.

Preheat the oven to 200°C/180°C fan/400°F/gas mark 6.

Wash and core the apples. Mix your chosen stuffing ingredients together in a small bowl with a fork and taste, then adjust the cinnamon and vanilla according to your liking. Push the stuffing into the cavities in the apples using your finger.

Put the apples into an ovenproof dish and cook for 20–30 minutes.

To make the vanilla custard, whisk the cornflour into 100ml (3½fl oz) of the milk in a mixing bowl until smooth. Soften the date in 3 tablespoons of the remaining milk either in a cup in the microwave for a minute or in a small pan over the heat, then mash with a fork. Put the purée into a sieve and push it through with the back of a spoon into the mixing bowl, then whisk into the cornflour mixture. Discard the skin of the date. Add the egg yolks to the bowl and whisk until smooth.

Heat the remaining milk and vanilla in a saucepan until very hot but not boiling. Whisk two ladlefuls of the hot milk into the egg mixture to equalize the temperature of the two liquids.

Now whisk the hot milk in the pan as you pour in the egg yolk mixture. Continue until thickened. Remove from the heat. If not using straight away, cover the surface with damp baking parchment to stop it forming a skin.

Remove the apples from the oven and serve with the custard or crème fraîche or mascarpone.

SERVES 4

4 cooking or eating apples, approx. 200g (7oz) each

For the spiced walnut stuffing

1 large Medjool date, pitted and chopped
60g (2¼oz) walnuts, chopped
60g (2¼oz) butter
1 teaspoon vanilla extract
1 teaspoon cinnamon or mixed spice

For the raspberry stuffing

1 large Medjool date, pitted and chopped
16 raspberries
1 teaspoon vanilla extract

For the vanilla custard (serves 6)

15g (½oz) cornflour
500ml (18fl oz) whole cow's or almond milk
1 large Medjool date, pitted and finely chopped
4 egg yolks
2 teaspoons vanilla extract

Per serving (walnut stuffing) 23g carbs, 4.2g fibre, 3g protein, 23g fat, 319kcal

Per serving (raspberry stuffing) 23g carbs, 4.4g fibre, 0.5g protein, 0.6g fat, 109kcal

Per serving of custard 8.9g carbs, 0.5g fibre, 4.9g protein, 6.9 g fat, 118kcal

Hot Raspberry Soufflé

This light and airy dessert isn't out of bounds, even on a sugar-free diet. We love the caramel flavour that the dates add to this, and it is plenty sweet enough if the raspberries are in season and ripe. If you are doing this in advance, say for a dinner party, prepare the raspberry custard until it is cooling in a bowl. Leave it in the fridge until you are ready, then beat it to get it smooth, as it will have set firm. Mix it with the egg whites as in the recipe.

Preheat the oven to 240°C/220°C fan/475°F/gas mark 9. Generously butter the insides and rims of 4 ramekins measuring about 9 x 4cm (3½ x 1½in).

Soften the chopped dates in 3 tablespoons of the milk either in a cup in the microwave for a minute or in a small pan over a low heat, then mash with a fork. Put the purée into a sieve over a bowl and push it through with the back of a spoon. Discard the skin of the dates.

Blitz the raspberries with a stick blender or food processor and sieve them into the date purée, discarding the seeds. Add the egg yolks and vanilla and stir to combine. Stir the cornflour into 3 tablespoons of the remaining milk in a small bowl until smooth then add this to the raspberry mixture.

Pour the remaining milk into a small saucepan and heat until very hot but not boiling. Pour a ladleful into your raspberry mixture, stir through, then add this to the pan and whisk until smooth. Continue to heat for a few minutes, stirring constantly over a medium heat, until it thickens. Remove from the heat and transfer the custard to a large bowl to cool for 10 minutes. Cover the surface with a piece of damp baking parchment to stop it forming a skin.

Meanwhile, whisk the egg whites in a large bowl with an electric whisk until they form soft peaks. Take a little of this mixture and use it to loosen the custard in the bowl. Whisk it to get rid of any lumps. Now, switch to a large metal spoon and gently fold in the remaining egg whites, keeping as much air in as possible. Spoon the mixture into the prepared ramekins and level the surface with a knife. Use the tip of your finger to wipe around the edge of each ramekin so that it is clean and the soufflé can rise easily. Stand the ramekins on a baking tray and bake for 8–10 minutes until risen and golden brown.

Heat the raspberry sauce in a small pan for a couple of minutes and transfer to a warm jug.

Remove the soufflés from the oven and serve straight away, decorated with the raspberries and hot raspberry sauce.

SERVES 4
a knob of butter, to grease
2 large Medjool dates
200ml (7fl oz) whole milk
200g (7oz) raspberries
4 eggs, separated
2 teaspoons vanilla extract
30g (1oz) cornflour

To serve
1 quantity of Raspberry Sauce
  (page 176)
12 raspberries

Per serving 24g carbs, 8.7g fibre, 11g protein, 27g fat, 406kcal

Chocolate, Coffee & Walnut Cake

Rich and decadent, this cake makes a delicious dessert. Choose a really dark, 85 per cent cocoa solids chocolate – with this amount of cocoa there isn't too much sugar in the chocolate. There will be some, but it will be minimal and you won't need any other sweetener. We have divided the cake into 12, which gives small slices, but it is filling because of the almonds, cream, butter and chocolate. A slice of chocolate cake made with sugar and flour can contain up to 40g carbs.

Preheat the oven to 190°C/170°C fan/375°F/gas mark 5. Line two 20cm (8in) round cake tins with baking parchment.

Melt the butter and chocolate together briefly in a bowl in the microwave; the best way to do this is to heat it in 30-second bursts so that you can keep an eye on it. Alternatively, pour a little hot water from a kettle into a small pan. Put a heatproof bowl over the pan, making sure the base doesn't touch the water. Put the butter and chocolate into the bowl and leave them to melt. Whisk them together to combine.

Grate the apples into a large mixing bowl (no need to peel). Add the remaining ingredients to the bowl and mix together thoroughly with a large spoon. Stir in the melted chocolate.

Spoon the mixture into the prepared tins, smooth the surface and bake for 20 minutes. Check that a cocktail stick comes out clean when inserted into the centre; if not, cook for a few minutes longer. Remove from the oven and allow to cool in the tins for a few minutes before removing and cooling on a wire rack.

To make the chocolate ganache, briefly heat the cream in a saucepan, and just before it boils, pour over the finely chopped dark chocolate in a bowl and stir through until you have a glossy, smooth ganache.

To assemble the cake, whip the cream with the vanilla extract until it forms soft peaks. Spread this on top of one of the cooled cakes. Put the other cake on top and spread over the ganache. Hold a cook's knife at a 45-degree angle to the remaining 25g (1oz) chocolate and scrape it into shavings, then scatter these on top. Serve straight away or keep chilled in the fridge for up to a day.

MAKES 1 CAKE/12 small portions

100g (3½oz) butter
100g (3½oz) dark (85%) chocolate, roughly chopped
2 dessert apples, approx. 200g (7oz) in total
70g (2½oz) walnuts or other nuts, roughly chopped
4 eggs
200g (7oz) ground almonds
1 tablespoon baking powder
1 tablespoon vanilla extract
4 tablespoons ground coffee (suitable for cafetières)

For the ganache

150ml (¼ pint) double cream
100g (3½oz) dark (85%) chocolate, 75g (2½oz) finely chopped and 25g (1oz) for shavings

For the filling

150ml (¼ pint) double cream
2 teaspoons vanilla extract

Per serving 9.4g carbs, 5.1g fibre, 9.7g protein, 43g fat, 491kcal

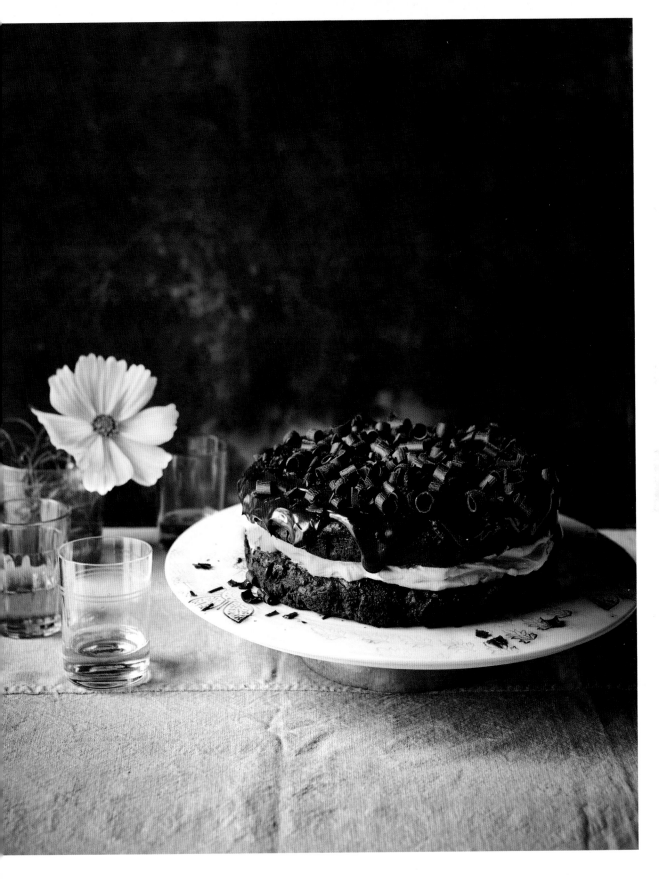

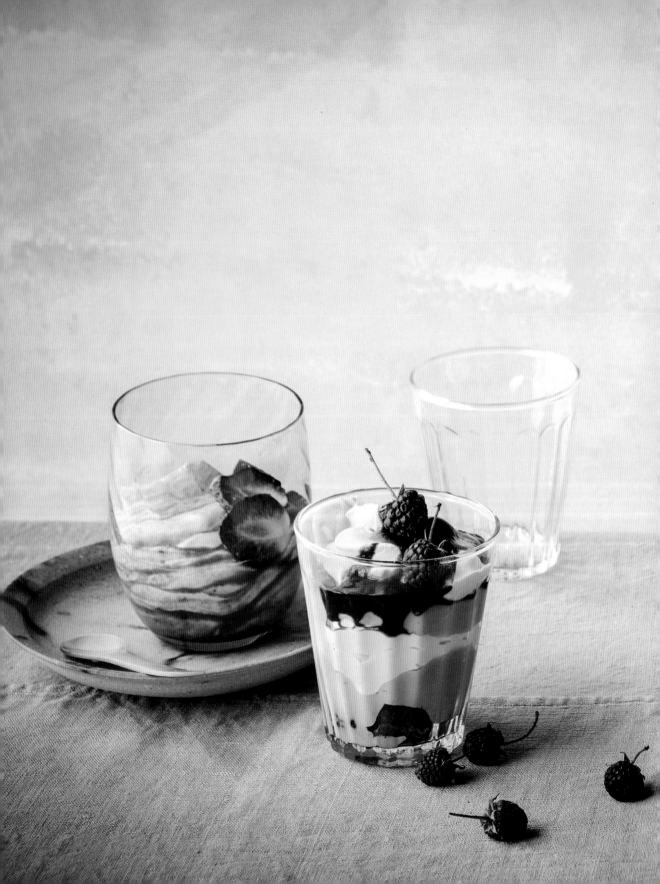

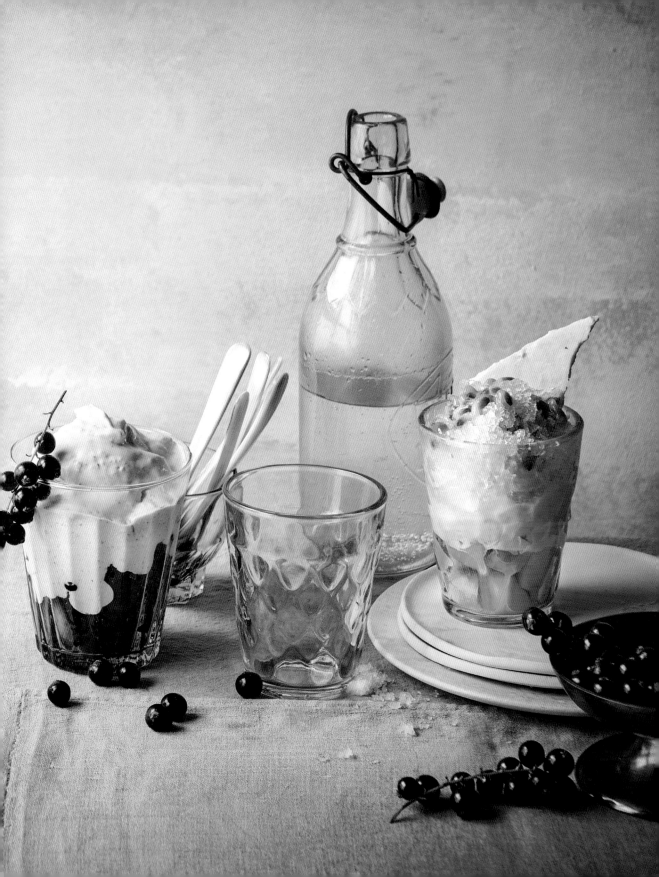

4 ways with... SUNDAES

Having grown up in Eastbourne, I was used to going to Romeo's, an Italian café near the seafront, and ordering huge ice-cream sundaes in tall conical glasses. They came with a long thin spoon to allow you to reach the pools of sweet strawberry sauce lurking at the bottom under the layers of canned fruit and vanilla ice cream. My taste might have moved away from ultra-sweet flavours, but I still love food with the wow factor and plenty of colour and texture differences.

From low-carb dairy, fruit, nuts and chocolate, you can create a wealth of delicious desserts without the sugar. Here we give some sundae suggestions but have also created a list so that you can have fun with flavour and texture. These sundaes are good for a quick pudding or for more glamorous entertaining. I have collected various glasses, from old hand-me-down champagne saucers to charity shop shot glasses. Don't feel they have to match; a random assortment is just as good.

Sundae Combinations

LOW-CARB FRUITS	FILLINGS	SAUCES	TOPPINGS
Peaches	Greek yogurt	Lemon curd	Toasted almonds
Raspberries	Whipped cream	Raspberry sauce	Chopped walnuts
Nectarines	Lemon Semifreddo	Chocolate sauce	Toasted coconut shavings
Strawberries	Whipped coconut cream	Strawberry jam	Chocolate shavings
Blueberries	Mascarpone		Coconut Ice-Cream Shards
Blackberries	Yogurt/cream mix		Roasted peanuts
Cooked apples	Vanilla custard		

Rhubarb & Strawberry Coulis Fool with Greek Yogurt & Whipping Cream

Naturally sweet strawberries offset the tartness of rhubarb and, helpfully, they grow at the same time in my garden. The creamy blend of natural yogurt and cream provides the perfect foil for the puréed fruit. Do swap the strawberries or rhubarb for other fruits; just purée and swirl into the cream.

For the purée, gently heat the ingredients together in a small pan for 15–20 minutes with the lid on, or until the fruit is soft. Transfer the mixture to a food processor or use a stick blender to make a purée. Chill in the fridge before use.

Whip the cream in a bowl until it forms soft peaks, then fold in the yogurt and vanilla extract. Swirl in the fruit purée and decant into small champagne saucers or flutes, or large shot glasses. Keep in the fridge for up to 2 days before serving chilled.

SERVES 6
225ml (8fl oz) whipping cream
225ml (8fl oz) Greek yogurt
1½ teaspoons vanilla extract

For the rhubarb and strawberry purée
225g (8oz) rhubarb, cleaned and roughly chopped
75g (2¾oz) strawberries, hulled and halved
50ml (2fl oz) water
2 Medjool dates, pitted and finely chopped

Per serving 13g carbs, 1.8g fibre, 5g protein, 17g fat, 271kcal

Frozen Berry Ice-cream Sundae

If you have fruit ready frozen, you can quickly assemble this low-carb ice-cream sundae. To keep the carbs down, for this recipe choose a banana that isn't too ripe or dark in colour. Peel, slice and freeze the banana. Hull and halve your strawberries before freezing – they will only need a few hours in a shallow dish. This works equally well with the Hot Chocolate Sauce from the Poached Pears recipe on page 178.

If there is room in your fridge or freezer, chill 6 small glasses.

Remove the frozen fruit from the freezer and immediately whizz in a food processor with the mascarpone. Blend just enough to break up the fruit but don't overwhip it or it will melt. (If this happens, put it back into the freezer to firm up.) Now assemble the sundaes by dividing the berries, raspberry sauce and ice cream between the glasses. Serve the chocolate sauce hot in a jug on the side.

SERVES 6
1 frozen sliced banana
125g (4½oz) frozen strawberries
250g (9oz) mascarpone
1 quantity of Raspberry Sauce (page 176)
200g (7oz) fresh berries, such as strawberries, raspberries, blackberries, blueberries or redcurrants

Per serving 10g carbs, 3.2g fibre, 2.8g protein, 19g fat, 230kcal

Lemon Curd, Raspberry & Cream Sundae

I love lemon curd, but it is usually laden with sugar. In this version we have used the natural sweetness of dates to take the edge off the sour lemon. It blends perfectly with the cream and raspberries to make a sundae. This delicious indulgence can be added once more to your diet as a treat, since we have invented a low-carb version of lemon curd. Do note that this should not be given to pregnant women or the elderly, though, as the eggs may not be sterilized. The raspberry sauce can also be made with fresh strawberries or blackberries. In this instance, you need the sauce cold, but it is delicious served hot over the Lemon Semifreddo on page 164 or the Frozen Berry Ice-cream Sundae on page 175.

Make the raspberry sauce by heating the raspberries with the vanilla extract in a small saucepan. Squash them with a potato masher and bring to the boil. Remove from the heat straight away and pour through a sieve to get rid of the pips. Allow to cool; cover and store in the fridge for up to 3 days.

To make the lemon curd, put the dates with the water and lemon juice into a small saucepan over a medium heat. Bring to a gentle boil, mashing the dates with a fork until they are puréed. Remove from the heat (reserve the pan) and sieve the mixture into a bowl, pushing the dates with the back of a spoon until only the skins remain in the sieve. Discard these.

Return the date purée to the saucepan and add the lemon zest and butter. The residual heat from the dates and saucepan should be enough to melt the butter. If not, put over a gentle heat, stirring to combine it. Remove the pan from the heat and quickly tip in the beaten egg yolks, stirring vigorously with a wooden spoon. When they are well combined, put the pan over a gentle heat once more and stir constantly until the curd just starts to thicken. Remove from the heat immediately and allow to cool. If not using straight away, store, covered, in the fridge for up to 3 days.

To assemble the sundae, whip the cream with the vanilla extract until it forms soft peaks. Divide the raspberries between 4 glasses, leaving a few to decorate the tops. Spoon an eighth of the lemon curd into each glass. Top with an eighth of the whipped cream, followed by the remaining lemon curd. Divide the remaining cream between the glasses then pour over the chilled raspberry sauce. Keep in the fridge until serving. They will keep for up to a day.

SERVES 4

200ml (7fl oz) whipping cream
1 teaspoon vanilla extract
120g (4¼oz) raspberries

For the raspberry sauce

150g (5½oz) frozen or fresh
  raspberries (or you can use fresh
  strawberries or blackberries)
1 teaspoon vanilla extract

For the lemon curd (makes 200g/7oz)

2 large Medjool dates, pitted and
  roughly chopped
4 tablespoons water
6 tablespoons lemon juice
  (approx. 2 large lemons)
finely grated zest of 1 lemon
70g (2½oz) butter
4 egg yolks, beaten

Per serving 14g carbs, 5.3g fibre, 5.2g protein, 40g fat, 464kcal
Lemon Curd (200g/7oz)
38g carbs, 5.3g fibre, 13g protein, 80g fat, 945kcal

Coconut & Lime Sundae with Tropical Fruit & Ice-cream Shards

Granita is a crunchy, granular sorbet from Sicily. On hot summer days, the fruit-flavoured ice is welcome and makes a popular dessert. This recipe uses the coconut water from a couple of chilled cans of coconut milk (as it separates when cold) to make the granita, and the coconut cream from the top to make a dairy-free whipped cream and ice-cream shards for the sundae. For an added kick, add 3 tablespoons of dark rum to the granita before freezing.

To make the granita, carefully spoon the coconut cream out of one chilled can of coconut milk and set aside for the coconut cream. Stir the remaining coconut water and vanilla together in a shallow bowl and put into the freezer for a couple of hours to set firm. When frozen, scrape the granita with a fork to form crystals. You can put it back into the freezer until you need it and it will keep, covered, for up to a month.

Whisk the coconut cream in a bowl with the vanilla for a couple of minutes until thick and firm. Leave in a cool place until you are ready to serve.

To assemble the sundaes, chill 6 small glasses in the fridge or freezer. Divide the mango, coconut granita and whipped coconut cream between the glasses. Scoop out the pulp and seeds from the passion fruit halves over the sundaes and top with the frozen coconut ice-cream shards. Serve straight away.

SERVES 6

3 passion fruits, halved
1 mango, cut into 2cm (¾in) chunks
Frozen Coconut Ice-cream Shards (below), to serve

For the coconut granita
400ml (14fl oz) coconut water from 2 x 400ml (14fl oz) cans of chilled coconut milk
1 teaspoon vanilla extract

For the whipped coconut cream
180–200g (6¼–7oz) coconut cream (from the top of a can or bought separately), chilled
1 teaspoon vanilla extract
finely grated zest of ½ lime

Per serving 11g carbs, 2.5g fibre, 2.2g protein, 24g fat, 276kcal

Frozen Coconut Ice-cream Shards
This is a great way to make quick ice-cream shapes from coconut cream.

180–200g (6¼–7oz) coconut cream (from the top of a can or bought separately), chilled
1 teaspoon vanilla extract

Put a small metal tray or a plate lined with a piece of baking parchment into your freezer to chill. Mix the coconut cream and vanilla extract together and spread onto the chilled, lined tray. Spread it out into a layer about 3mm (⅛in) thick. Return the tray to the freezer and let the cream set firm. Peel away the paper from the back of the frozen sheet of coconut cream and break into shards. Return to the freezer quickly until you are ready to serve.

Poached Pears with Orange Stuffing & Hot Chocolate Sauce

These pretty pears can be prepared in advance and stored in the fridge until you are ready to serve. I like to serve them chilled from the fridge with a jug of hot chocolate sauce to pour over the top.

Peel the pears, leaving the stalks intact, and put them into a medium-size pan with enough hot water to cover them. Add the lemon juice and squeezed lemon halves, cinnamon stick and vanilla and bring to the boil. Cover the pan and cook the pears until tender. Ripe ones only need about 15 minutes but unripe, firm pears may need up to 1 hour. Pierce them with a skewer or fork to check they are soft.

Meanwhile, make the stuffing by mixing the ingredients together into a paste in a small bowl, mashing the date to distribute it evenly. Set aside.

Remove the cooked pears from the pan using a slotted spoon and stand them on a serving plate to cool to room temperature. Slice off the top 3cm (1¼in) of each pear and reserve. Carefully cut out the centres using an apple corer. Use a teaspoon and your finger to push the stuffing into the cavities. Put the tops back on the pears.

When you are ready to serve, stand the pears onto individual plates. To make the chocolate sauce, heat the cream to just below boiling in a small pan. Pour over the chocolate in a bowl and stir through until you have a glossy, smooth sauce. Spoon over the pears before serving or serve it separately in a warm jug.

SERVES 4

4 medium, ripe pears
juice of 1 lemon (put the squeezed
*   halves in the water in which you*
*   cook the pears)*
5cm (2in) cinnamon stick
1 teaspoon vanilla extract

For the stuffing
50g (1¾oz) full-fat cream cheese
finely grated zest of ½ orange
1 Medjool date, pitted and
*   chopped finely*

For the hot chocolate sauce
125ml (4fl oz) double cream
50g (1¾oz) dark (85%) chocolate,
*   finely chopped*

Per serving 28g carbs, 6.2g fibre, 2.9g protein, 27g fat, 372kcal

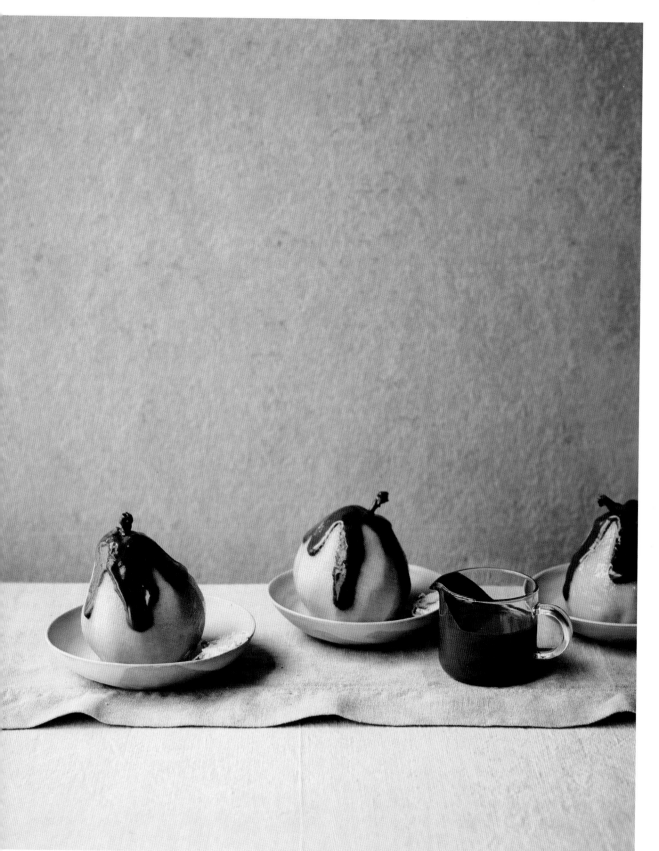

Tiramisu

We have been making tiramisu for years in our restaurants, but as soon as we decided to cut our carb intake, we had to come up with a new way to enjoy this glorious Italian classic. Stefano Borella, expert pastry chef and head teacher at our cookery school, has been experimenting for months to perfect this version and it halves the carbs of a typical tiramisu. We have used dates to add sweetness and a wonderful caramel flavour to the cream.

As we are encouraging people to have small servings of desserts, we suggest using old champagne saucers, small tumblers or large shot glasses – if they are big enough to hold 100ml (3½fl oz) of water, which is the right size for the tiramisu. Alternatively, make one tiramisu in a dish about 25 x 20cm (10 x 8in). Do note that this should not be given to pregnant women or the elderly, as the eggs are not cooked.

Preheat the oven to 190°C/170°C fan/375°F/gas mark 5 and line a 20cm (8in) round cake tin with baking parchment.

Soften the dates in the very hot water in a mug, mashing them with a fork. Use a spoon to push the softened dates through a sieve into a bowl, discarding the skins. Add the egg yolks and vanilla and whisk together. Sift in the ground almonds and baking powder and stir to combine.

In another bowl, whisk the egg whites with clean, dry beaters until they hold the shape of stiff peaks. Now gently fold the egg whites into the egg yolk mixture with a large spoon just until the mixture is all one colour. Pour this mixture into the cake tin and put into the oven for 18–20 minutes or until firm to the touch and lightly browned. Remove the cake from the tin and allow to cool on a wire rack.

Cut the sponge into finger-size pieces and set aside.

To make the cream, soften the date in the very hot water in a mug, mashing it with a fork. Use a spoon to push the softened date through a sieve into a mixing bowl, discarding the skin. Add the mascarpone, egg yolks and vanilla and use an electric mixer, or hand whisk, to whisk the mixture until well combined and creamy. Whip the whipping cream until it forms soft peaks and gently fold into the mascarpone mixture.

Whisk the egg whites with clean, dry beaters until they form soft peaks and lightly fold into the cream mixture.

Mix the coffee and marsala together in a small bowl. Dip the sponge fingers briefly into the liquid and divide them between the glasses. Divide the cream between 8 glasses and chill in fridge for at least an hour and up to 24 hours. Serve dusted with sifted cocoa powder.

SERVES 8

For the sponge

3 large Medjool dates, pitted and finely chopped
2 tablespoons very hot water
3 eggs, separated
1 teaspoon vanilla extract
75g (2¾oz) ground almonds
1 teaspoon baking powder

For the cream

1 large Medjool date, pitted and finely chopped
2 tablespoons very hot water
200g (7oz) mascarpone
150ml (¼ pint) whipping cream
2 eggs, separated
1 teaspoon vanilla extract

To serve

100ml (3½fl oz) cold strong coffee
3 tablespoons Marsala, brandy or Amaretto
2 tablespoon cocoa powder, to dust

Per serving 12g carbs, 2.6g fibre, 8.5g protein, 27g fat, 333kcal

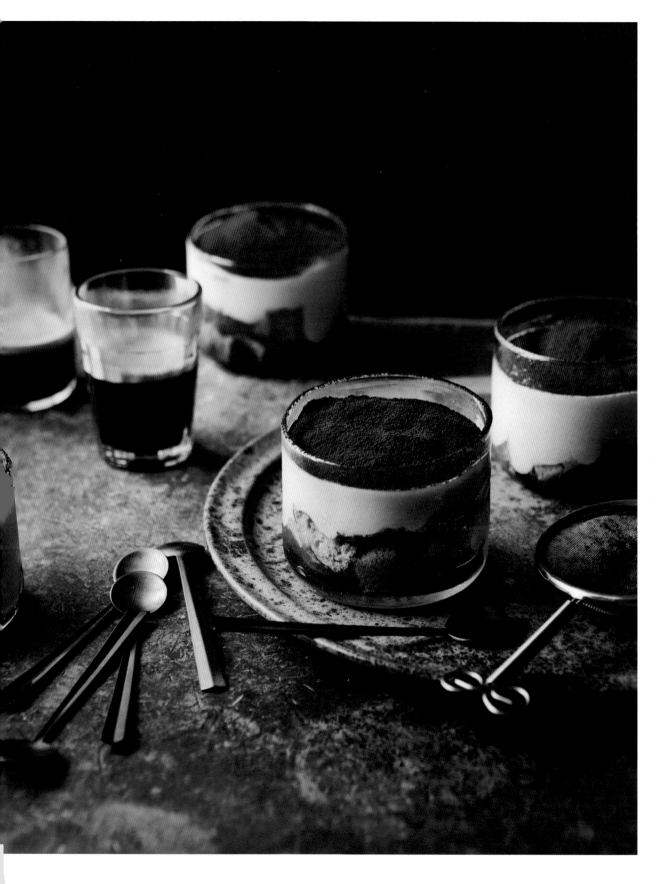

Apple, Carrot & Walnut Loaf with Cream Cheese Frosting

This easy-to-make, versatile loaf cake is perfect on its own with a cup of coffee, spread with butter and the Sicilian Clementine Marmalade on page 185 for breakfast or dressed up with a cream cheese frosting for tea.

Preheat the oven to 200°C/180°C fan/400°F/gas mark 6. Generously butter and line a 650g (1lb 7oz) loaf tin with baking parchment. Put the pecans on a small baking tray and cook for 8–10 minutes to brown. Remove from the oven and leave to cool. Chop the nuts roughly and set aside.

Mash the date into the very hot water in a large mixing bowl using a fork to form a paste. Add the grated carrot and apples to the bowl, then the remaining ingredients and mix together thoroughly with a large spoon.

Spoon into the prepared tin, level the surface and bake for 45 minutes. Check that a cocktail stick comes out clean when inserted into the centre; if not, cook for a few minutes longer. Remove from the oven and leave to cool in the tin for 5 minutes. Turn out of the tin and leave to cool completely on a wire rack before serving.

Make up the frosting by beating the orange zest into the cream cheese in a bowl, then stir in the vanilla and milk. Spread it on top of the cooled cake and scatter over the nuts.

SERVES 10

100g (3½oz) butter or coconut oil, melted, plus a little extra to grease
2 Medjool dates, pitted and roughly chopped
2 tablespoons very hot water
1 carrot, approx. 120g (4½oz), coarsely grated
2 medium apples, peeled, cored and coarsely grated
25g (1oz) ground flaxseed
50g (1¾oz) coconut flour
4 eggs, beaten
100g (3½oz) ground almonds
2 heaped teaspoons gluten-free baking powder
1 tablespoon vanilla extract
2 teaspoons mixed spice

For the topping

½ teaspoon finely grated orange zest
180g (6¼oz) full-fat cream cheese
1 teaspoon vanilla extract
2 tablespoons milk
50g (1½oz) pecans or walnuts, cut into slivers

Per serving 11g carbs, 4.9g fibre, 8.1g protein, 25g fat, 308kcal

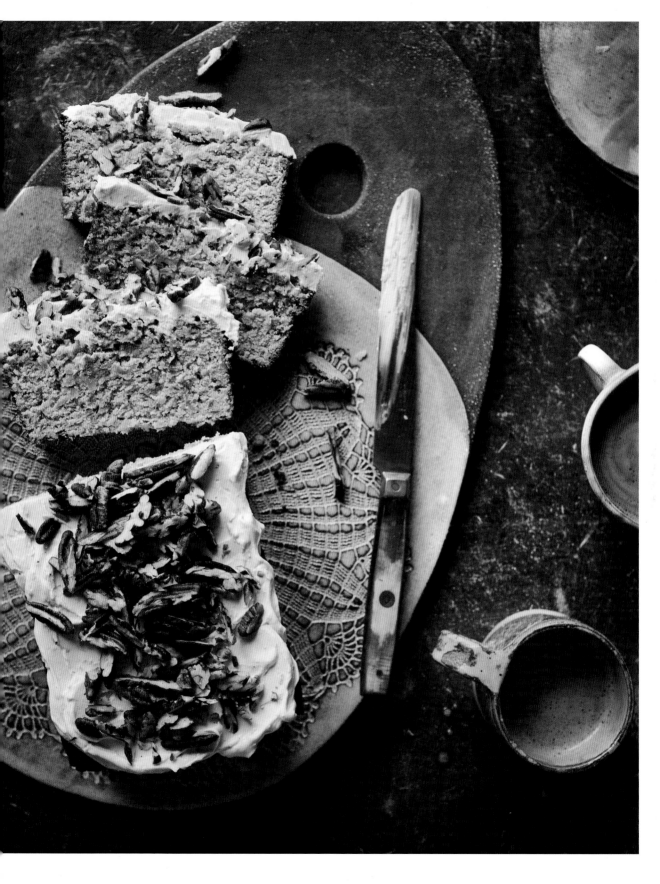

Coconut & Lemon Cake

Sweet coconut cake meets sharp lemon curd in a cloud of whipped cream in this impressive celebration cake. The clever part is that the egg whites lighten the cake, while the leftover yolks make the velvety lemon curd. The cake and the curd can be made and stored, covered, in the fridge a couple of days before you need them. Use any seasonal low-carb berries to top the cake or leave it with just the cream.

Preheat the oven to 190°C/170°C fan/375°F/gas mark 5. Grease a 20cm (8in) round cake tin generously with butter and line the base with a circle of baking parchment.

Soften the date in 3 tablespoons of the milk in a small bowl in a microwave – it will take about 30 seconds on full heat. Alternatively, heat it in a small pan over a medium heat. Mash it with a fork until you have a purée. Set aside to cool.

Put the ground almonds, coconut, coconut flour and baking powder in a large mixing bowl and combine with a fork. Add the melted butter, vanilla extract and lemon zest and stir through. Sieve the date purée into the bowl, discarding the skins. Add the remaining milk and stir through.

Beat the egg whites in a bowl with an electric whisk until they form stiff peaks. Use the whisk to beat a little of the egg whites into the cake batter to loosen it. Then switch to a large metal spoon and fold in the remaining egg whites. Be gentle and don't overmix it.

Spoon the batter into the prepared tin and bake for 25–30 minutes or until golden brown and a cocktail stick inserted into the centre comes out clean. Remove from the oven and leave to cool in the tin for 15 minutes. Run a round-bladed knife around the edge to loosen the cake before carefully turning it out onto a wire rack. When the cake has cooled to room temperature it can be transferred to a serving dish.

Use a spatula to spread the cake with a generous layer of lemon curd (if you feel it is too much, the remainder will always keep in the fridge for a couple of days). Whip the cream in a bowl with an electric whisk until soft peaks form and spoon over the cake. Top with the berries and serve straight away or chill in the fridge for a few hours.

SERVES 8

100g (3½oz) butter, melted, plus extra to grease
1 Medjool date, pitted and roughly chopped
150ml (¼ pint) whole milk
100g (3½oz) ground almonds
100g (3½oz) unsweetened desiccated coconut
35g (1¼oz) coconut flour
1 heaped teaspoon gluten-free baking powder
2 teaspoons vanilla extract
finely grated zest of 1 large lemon
4 egg whites (reserve the yolks for the lemon curd)

To serve

1 quantity of Lemon Curd (page 176)
150ml (¼ pint) whipping cream
150g (5½oz) berries, such as strawberries, raspberries or blueberries

Per serving 10g carbs, 3.9g fibre, 7.9g protein, 36g fat, 407kcal

Peanut Butter Cookies

Nut butters are full of good fats, and because of their high fibre content, they will fill you up until the next meal. Take them to work or allow yourself one after a meal to satiate any sugar cravings.

Preheat the oven to 190°C/170°C fan/375°F/gas mark 5. Line a baking tray with baking parchment or a silicone mat. Soften the dates in the water in a mug, using a fork to mash them to a purée. Add the purée to a large mixing bowl with the rest of the ingredients, except the raspberries or chocolate. Combine using a metal spoon.

Form into walnut-size balls, then place, spaced apart, on the prepared baking tray and flatten each one slightly to about 5cm (2in) in diameter. Make a small indent in the centre of each with your fingertip. Pop a raspberry (domed side up) or a piece of chocolate on top of each one. Bake for 10–12 minutes or until lightly browned. Remove from the oven and allow to cool on the tray before storing in an airtight container for up to 3 days.

MAKES 20–25 BISCUITS

*2 Medjool dates, pitted and
  roughly chopped
2 tablespoons very hot water
200g (7oz) peanut butter
200g (7oz) ground almonds
25g (1oz) ground flaxseeds
2 medium eggs
1 tablespoon vanilla extract
2 teaspoons baking powder
pinch of salt if the peanut butter
  isn't salted
25 raspberries or 10g (¼ oz) 85%
  dark chocolate, broken into
  small (pea-size) pieces*

Per serving 3.1g carbs, 2.7g fibre, 5.8g protein, 11g fat, 139kcal

Sicilian Clementine Marmalade

We discovered this soft-set marmalade in Sicily where naturally sweet clementines don't need any added sugar. It keeps in the fridge for a month and is lovely on the Apple, Carrot & Walnut Loaf on page 182 or with mascarpone on the toasted Flaxseed Bread Rolls on page 101.

Put the clementines and apple into a saucepan with the hot water and bring to the boil. Reduce the heat to low and cook for 1 hour, stirring frequently until the flesh is very soft and squashes easily with a spoon against the side of the pan. Mash the dates to a purée with the very hot water using a fork, then push through a sieve using the back of a spoon into the simmering marmalade, discarding the skins. Add the vanilla extract. The marmalade will lose water as it cooks and concentrate to a thick jammy consistency. It will be loose set, so you don't need to do anything other than decide how thick you want it and stop the cooking when it is ready. Taste, and if you find it too bitter, add another puréed date.

Pour just-boiled water from a kettle into your jam jars and over the lids to clean them. Use tongs to tip the water out and let them dry. Fill the still-warm jars with the hot marmalade and put on the lids. Allow to cool and put into the fridge. Consume within a month.

MAKES APPROX. 650G (1lb 7oz) or 3 small jam jars

*500g (1lb 2oz) clementines,
  washed and stalks removed,
  chopped into 1cm (½in) pieces
1 medium apple, cored and
  chopped into 1cm (½in) pieces
400ml (14fl oz) hot water
2 large Medjool dates, pitted and
  roughly chopped
3 tablespoons very hot water
1 teaspoon vanilla extract*

Per 30g serving 6.1g carbs, 0.7g fibre, 0.5g protein, 0g fat, 29kcal

6 ways with... DRINKS

The downfall of most drinks is what you have with them rather than the alcohol alone. However, going low-carb can mean that you are more affected by alcohol because you are carrying less water in your body, so go easy, as you might find less is more.

Pure spirits, such as gin, tequila, brandy, whisky and vodka, don't have a carb value, but when you want a long drink, what do you do? Here are some suggestions that won't have you opening the artificially sweetened or sugary mixers.

Champagne, dry whites and red wines are good options to drink, as they are low in carbs but in recent years, I find I am affected by sulphite, which is added to some wines to prevent oxidation. To know that you are consuming a purer product with fewer added chemicals, choose natural, low-intervention wines. They will probably be labelled organic, biodynamic or vegan, but it is best to speak to a wine dealer who can advise on low-sulphite wines. I like to find fruity reds and, during summer, I drink them chilled. I also do as the Italians and French do: never drink on an empty stomach. Instead, accompany wine as an aperitif with olives and salumi.

Strawberry Daiquiri

Here are some suggestions worked out, shaken and stirred by our son Giorgio that won't have you opening the artificially sweetened or sugary mixers. This is best made when strawberries are in season and full of natural sweetness. It can also be made with raspberries. Despite their sweet nature, these berries are low in carbohydrates, so you can feel good about the odd daiquiri on a hot summer's evening.

Put the strawberries with the rum, lime juice, vanilla and ice into a small food processor and whizz to a purée. Serve straight away in a chilled glass with the extra strawberry and slice of lime.

MAKES 1 COCKTAIL

80g (2¾oz) fresh strawberries, washed and hulled, plus 1 whole strawberry, to serve
60ml (4 tablespoons) rum
juice of ¼ lime
¼ teaspoon vanilla
50g (1¾oz) ice
1 slice of lime, to finish

Per serving 4.9g carbs, 3g fibre, 0.5g protein, 0.5g fat, 167kcal

Frozen Raspberry Daiquiri

This is a good all-year-round cocktail, as frozen raspberries are always readily available.

Put the frozen raspberries, ice, rum, vanilla, and lime juice into a small food processor and whizz to a purée. Pour into a chilled glass. Put the mint in the palm of your hand and clap your other hand onto it – this lightly bruises it to release the aroma. Sit the bruised mint on top of the cocktail and enjoy straight away.

MAKES 1 COCKTAIL

80g (2¾oz) frozen raspberries
50g (1¾oz) ice
60ml (4 tablespoons) rum
½ teaspoon vanilla extract
juice of ¼ lime
1 sprig of mint, to finish

Per serving 4g carbs, 5.7g fibre, 1g protein, 0.5g fat, 173kcal

Cava Roja

As long as you buy a dry (brut) sparkling wine, then you can use prosecco, cava or champagne for this cocktail, as they are all low in carbs. Normally, the fruit syrups added to cocktails are loaded with sugar, but by using ripe low-carb berries and vanilla extract you don't need any sweeteners.

Make the sauce by heating the raspberries in a small saucepan over a medium heat. Cook them for just 5 minutes then use a potato masher to squash the fruit into a pulpy sauce. Pass the purée through a fine-mesh sieve into a jug to remove the pips.

To make the cocktail, put the raspberry sauce into the bottom of a champagne flute or saucer. Top up with the cava and give it a gentle stir with a long spoon or fork to distribute the sauce. Serve straight away.

MAKES I COCKTAIL
For the raspberry sauce
150g (5½oz) raspberries, fresh or frozen
1 teaspoon vanilla extract

For 1 cocktail
2 tablespoons raspberry sauce (above)
100ml (3½fl oz) cava brut

Per serving 2.9g carbs, 1.9g fibre, 0.5g protein, 0g fat, 24kcal

Whisky Highball

Our son Giorgio and I loved this on our travels in Japan. It is a refreshing way to drink your favourite whisky, and opens up the flavours as well as making it into a long drink. Use the whisky of your choice; we like Japanese whisky that isn't smoky or peaty, but the choice is yours. You will be pleased to know that whisky and other clear spirits don't contain carbs.

Pour the whisky into a glass filled with ice, squeeze in the lemon juice and drop in the wedge. Top up with the soda water.

SERVES 1
60ml (4 tablespoons) whisky
ice
¼ lemon to squeeze, plus a wedge of lemon to serve
70ml (2½fl oz) soda water, to top up

Per serving 0.5g carbs, 0g fibre, 0g protein, 0g fat, 136kcal

Summer Sangria

A good fruity sangria is a delicious drink on a hot day but is usually loaded with added sugar or lemonade. It doesn't need either, as the natural sweetness of the fruit is enough. I like to use Nero d'Avola, a red from Sicily, but a Merlot or a Cabernet Sauvignon is also good; do chill the bottle first. This is the basic recipe below but, depending what is in season, add other fruit, such as strawberries, slices of peach or nectarine, or a few sprigs of mint to serve as you like.

Put the fruit into a large jug and add the orange juice and brandy. Use a wooden spoon to press the fruit a little so that the flavours muddle. Now pour in the chilled red wine and allow the flavours to mingle for 15 minutes or up to 1 hour in the fridge.

Serve over ice in large glasses topped up with soda water to taste and any additional sliced fruit.

SERVES 8–10

1 apple, cored and cut into 2cm (¾in) cubes
2 oranges, 1 cut into slices, the other juiced
125ml (4fl oz) brandy
75cl bottle fruity red wine, such as Nero d'Avola, chilled
ice, to serve
1 -litre (2¾-pint) bottle soda water

Per serving 4.9g carbs, 0.6g fibre, 0.6g protein, 0g fat, 130kcal

Mulled Wine

A cold winter night's version of the summer sangria, this mulled wine is warming and makes your house smell Christmassy and traditional. I suggest making this without any honey, but to please a crowd, add the minimum amount, just to take the edge off any bitterness. It will still be a lot less sugar-heavy than traditional mulled wine.

Put everything into a large saucepan over a low heat for 15 minutes or until piping hot. Don't let it boil or you will burn away the alcohol.

Use a ladle to transfer into heatproof glasses, making sure everyone has a little fruit in their glass.

SERVES 8–10

3 long strips of orange zest, all white pith discarded
1 apple, cored and cut into 2cm (¾in) cubes
a thumb-sized knob of ginger, peeled and sliced
1 cinnamon stick
1 star anise
juice of 1 orange
125ml (4fl oz) brandy
75cl bottle fruity red wine, such as Merlot
400ml (14fl oz) water, to taste
2 teaspoons mild honey

Per serving 4.8g carbs, 0.5g fibre, 0.5g protein, 0g fat, 128kcal

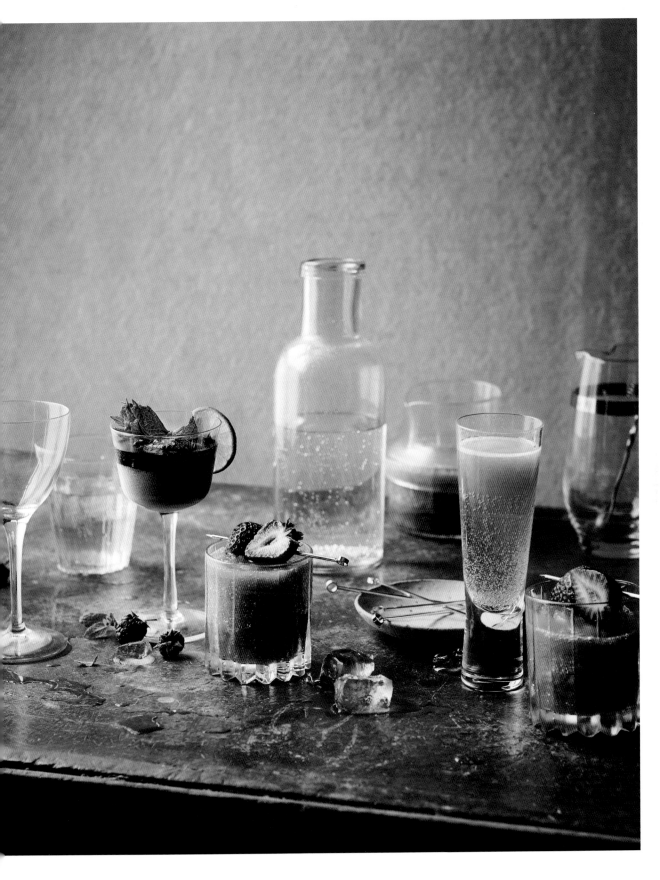

Resources & References

Primarily we used www.nutritics.com for the nutritional analysis.

Diabetes.co.uk, the global diabetes community.

www.lowcarbprogram.com is a digital program that redefines metabolic health.

Carbs & Cals produce carb and calorie counter books and apps.

Freestyle Libre makes instant glucose monitoring systems and can be found at www.freestylelibre.co.uk.

The Public Health Collaboration is a charity dedicated to informing and implementing decisions for better public health. Find out more at www.phcuk.org.

See www.westonaprice.org for information nutrition and health.

See www.dietdoctor.com for information on low-carb diets.

For a list of scientific references please go to www.inspirednutrition.co.uk

Acknowledgements

Giancarlo, Jenny and I were delighted to work with Dr David Unwin and Dr Jen Unwin on this project. Their knowledge, experience and help were invaluable. We wish it to be known that they have received no fee for their participation in this book. Instead we made a donation to the Public Health Collaboration to further their work spreading the real food message.

Massive thanks to Anna Hudson, Clare Gray, Stefano Borella, Liz Bentham, Carol Bradley, Aubrey Allen Butchers, Devin from Savannah Butchers in Gerrards Cross and Claire Smith.

Thank you to Vicky Orchard, editor, and Allison Gonsalves in production as well as our agent Jonathan Hayden. The book is beautiful thanks to Maja Smend for the photography and Susie Theodorou, Evie and Nicole for the styling and props.

Thank you for the Japanese inspiration from Cooking Sun Cookery School in Kyoto, Atsushi and Mayumi Momose in Nagano and the Aoki family in Sendai.

To my oldest friends – Karin Piper, Tanya Montgomery and Judy Knapp – sorry for making you cook all weekend when we should have been on the beach!

And to our lovely sons – that is the end of the washing up and yes, you can have what you want now, not just what is in the fridge and needs eating up!

Find Katie and Giancarlo at www.caldesi.com, on Instagram and Twitter @katiecaldesi, Facebook under Caldesi Italian Restaurants. Dr David Unwin @lowcarbGP, Dr Jen Unwin @jen_unwin and/or @realfoodrocksUK, Jenny Phillips on twitter @jennynutrition and www.inspirednutrition.co.uk

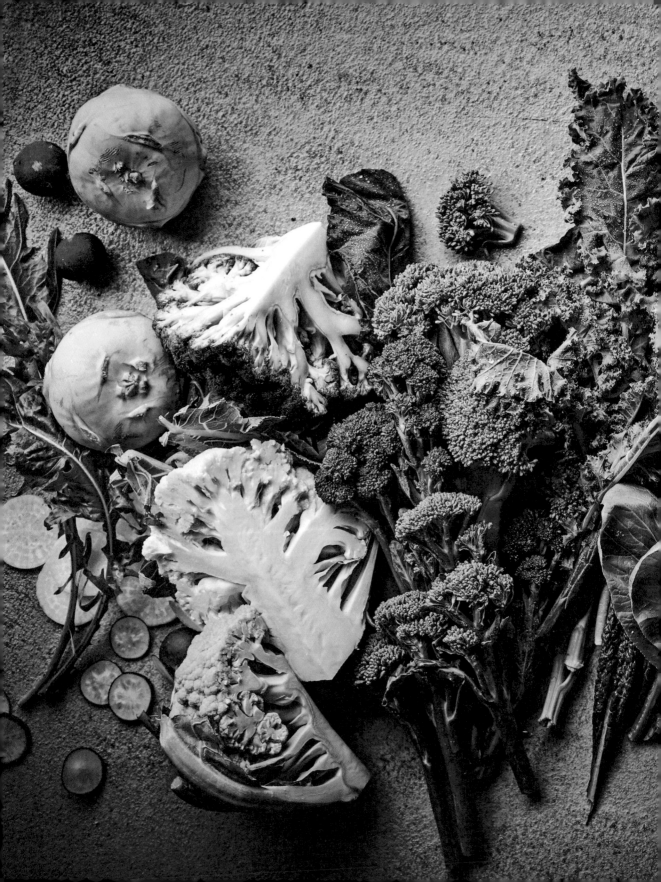